THE PHYSIOLOGY OF CARTILAGINOUS, FIBROUS, AND BONY TISSUE

THE PHYSIOLOGY OF CARTILAGINOUS, FIBROUS, AND BONY TISSUE

By

HAROLD M. FROST, M.D.,
A.O.A., A.A.O.S., A.B.J.S.

*Chairman
Department of Orthopaedic Surgery
Henry Ford Hospital
Detroit, Michigan*

*Orthopaedic Lectures
Volume II*

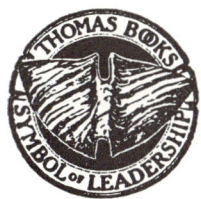

CHARLES C THOMAS • PUBLISHER
Springfield • Illinois • U.S.A.

Published and Distributed Throughout the World by
CHARLES C THOMAS • PUBLISHER
BANNERSTONE HOUSE
301-327 East Lawrence Avenue, Springfield, Illinois, U.S.A.

This book is protected by copyright. No part of it may be reproduced in any manner without written permission from the publisher.

© 1972, by CHARLES C THOMAS • PUBLISHER
ISBN 0-398-02562-2
Library of Congress Catalog Card Number: 72-79189

With THOMAS BOOKS *careful attention is given to all details of manufacturing and design. It is the Publisher's desire to present books that are satisfactory as to their physical qualities and artistic possibilities and appropriate for their particular use.* THOMAS BOOKS *will be true to those laws of quality that assure a good name and good will.*

Printed in the United States of America
JJ-23

Preface

This series of monographs has a *principal target:* practicing physicians and their residents who must deal clinically with skeletal problems, whether by medical, orthotic, surgical, or other means.

They have a *principal objective:* to translate into clinically useful concepts and language some of the meaning in terms of function, growth, and disease of behavioral relationships found in normal and diseased skeletal tissues. Herein, the term "skeletal tissues" will signify those appearing in the bony, articular, ligamentous, fascial, and tendonous parts of the body.

In pursuit of that objective, the monographs deliberately emphasize and deemphasize things in ways that may appear foreign to some "pure" basic scientists for the following reasons.

During part of my professional life I manage an active orthopaedic surgical practice and help to train orthopaedic residents, both of which activities acquaint me with problems peculiar both to the clinic and to teaching residents how to make clinical use of their basic science knowledge.

In the remainder of my professional life I do skeletal physiological research. Now, anyone who wears those particular "hats" has a unique opportunity to peer, with the awareness and insight peculiar to one, into the knowledge and expertise of the other, and to detect thereby utilitarian value and potential unrecognized by those who work wholly and only within either field.

Such insight exposed me, as a clinician, to some of the basic science explosions that occurred in this century, which have given us new analytical and investigative tools of great power. These tools include more than sophisticated instrumentation and machinery and precise measurement of subtle physical and chemical phenomena: they also include *purely conceptual approaches to studying physiological problems.* Physicians have been so inundated by patients that they have had no time to learn to exploit such conceptual advances systematically. For example, who among you know the contributions of medical value made by C. E. Shannon,[83] Norbert Wiener,[101] Watson and Crick, Uspensky, J. M. Reiner,[75] Paul Weiss,[100] F. Jacob and J. Monod,[49] or d'Arcy Thompson? Do not feel "put down" if these names ring no familiar bells in your mind, because while others read about them you were helping dozens of sick patients.

With respect to the division between clinic and laboratory, the intellectual approaches, jargon, and even the psychology required to function effectively and competently in each of these areas of endeavor differ so greatly that an interested person on one side cannot acquaint himself with the expertise of the other simply by asking. While it may seem ridiculous, nevertheless, total mutual misunderstanding usually frustrates such attempts; the basic scientist might as well address the physician in ancient Greek and have the latter reply in Mary Sherman's favorite second tongue, Hopi. Disturbing, pathetic, comical, frustrating: this situation is all of these and still more.

So, this text, addressed to clinicians and their residents, attempts to enhance their clinical perceptiveness and versatility by translating and forging into utilitarian implements what have too long remained strictly laboratory phenomena, insufficiently applied to clinical problems simply because the highly qualified basic scientists who understand them best have insufficient knowledge of clinical matters to realize where their expertise bears on it and where it does not. While serendipity (i.e. blind luck) has led to measureable progress in that regard, we must and—as Chapters IX and X promise—can do far better in the future. Thus, I hope that people highly qualified in some of the basic science aspects touched on herein will make due allowance if, on occasion, they find that the "translation" lacks the rigor, inclusiveness, emphasis, jargon, and/or depth they expect to find among their own colleagues.

The text does omit many things: detailed consideration of teeth, elastic cartilage, biomechanics per se, hematopoietic activity, biochemistry, and genetics; it omits them partly for reasons of space, because others have better qualifications for writing about them, because nobody yet knows enough about some of them to discuss them in a clinically meaningful way, and because some of them receive attention in later volumes of this series. The text contains a relatively small bibliography, because to do justice to that problem would require listing far more than 1000 references.

Finally, an apology, albeit a rather feeble one: I regret that the pure clinician (to whom the book is addressed) may well find some of this difficult to grasp the first time around because it presents familiar phenomena from unaccustomed viewpoints and in the focus of unfamiliar concepts. Exactly the absence of those concepts, however, makes clinical orthopaedics of today still largely a distillate of empirical, trial-and-error experiences accumulated over more than 2000 years of the history of man. If we would progress any faster in the next 2000 years than we did in the last, exactly those concepts *must* enter into everyday clinical work. So, granting that these efforts may contain many imperfections, accept my assurance based on over two decades of my own experience that they may also contain much merit, and let us now have a go at it.

HAROLD M. FROST

Acknowledgments

Many people have made these volumes possible, and it gives me pleasure to identify them here.

Teachers and mentors: J. W. O'Meara, F. N. Potts, B. E. Obletz, J. D. Godfrey, J. Talbot, O. Herzberg, D. M. Bosworth, B. Andrews, C. O. Bechtol, C. L. Mitchell, R. Buerki, F. R. Thompson, W. A. Armstrong, F. C. McLean, Randal Payne, N. Scatcherd, and H. Boyd.

Colleagues: P. A. Casagrande, A. Haddad, T. Rob, J. L. Fleming, D. C. Mitchell, C. White, L. Z. Shifrin, E. R. Guise, R. H. Ramsey, H. Pedersen, H. Duncan, B. Frame, R. A. Arnstein, B. N. Epker, E. Sedlin, S. Stanisavljevic, R. Wilson, T. Rush, L. Ilnicki, R. Hattner, H. Takahashi, O. Landeros, L. C. Johnson, J. S. Arnold, W. S. S. Jee, M. R. Urist, and Wm. Fielding.

Other assistants: R. R. Villanueva, D. B. Smith, J. Gray, R. Mohr, B. Hentschel. And my ever loving, long-suffering parents.

Institutions: Worchester City Hospital, Yale University School of Medicine, Buffalo General Hospital and Childrens Hospital, Henry Ford Hospital.

H.M.F.

CONTENTS

	Page
Preface	v
Acknowledgments	ix

Chapter

I.	Lectures in Skeletal Physiology	3
II.	The Basic Functional Plan of the Skeleton	23
III.	Histogenesis of Simple Skeletal Tissues	43
IV.	Histogenesis of Complex Skeletal Tissues	83
V.	The Endochondral Ossification Process	103
VI.	Biomechanical Responses of Hyaline Chondral Growth	120
VII.	Clinical Application of the Chondral Modeling Laws	140
VIII.	Biomechanical Response Characteristics of Fibrous Tissue	165
IX.	An Optimizing Strategy for Medical Research	185
X.	Application of Strategy	205

Bibliography	229
Answers to Questions	235
Glossary	243
Index	247

PREVIOUS PUBLICATIONS BY THE AUTHOR

Clinical Fundamentals of Orthopaedic Surgery, Grune and Stratton, New York, 1953 (Coauthored with P. A. Casagrande).

Bone Remodelling Dynamics, Springfield, Thomas, 1963.

Mathematical Elements of Lamellar Bone Remodeling, Springfield, Thomas, 1964.

The Laws of Bone Structure, Springfield, Thomas, 1964.

Bone Biodynamics, Boston, Little, Brown and Co., 1964 (Chief editor and contributor).

Clinical Orthopaedics, Vol. 49, 1966 (Guest editor of Symposium volume).

An Introduction to Biomechanics, Springfield, Thomas, 1966.

Bone Dynamics in Osteoporosis and Osteomalacia, Springfield, Thomas, 1966.

Orthopaedic Lecture Series: Vol. I, Surgery of Spasticity, Springfield, Thomas, 1972.

THE PHYSIOLOGY OF CARTILAGINOUS, FIBROUS, AND BONY TISSUE

Chapter I

Lectures in Skeletal Physiology

For later use, this chapter defines the meanings and/or workings of systems, systems analyses, functions, control system, feedback. It also defines the relation of the later textual content to the levels of biological organization lying between the cell and the man.

INTRODUCTION

Orthopaedic residents repeatedly expose (to any with eyes to see it) their great desire, not for knowledge as such but rather to understand. Of course, little difficulty arises in trying to understand the mechanical forces that caused a fracture-dislocation of some joint, or in trying to understand the therapeutically applied forces that will reduce it. Difficulty does arise when one looks at an x-ray of a deformed child and attempts to deduce what caused the deformities; when one looks at a microscopic slide of a bone lesion and tries to deduce the basic nature of the process it represents, as well as what preprinted label (otherwise known as the diagnosis) to paste on it; or when one wants to devise a corrective treatment for some deformity which, for whatever reason, fails to follow a standard course.

Our residents correctly tend to value understanding above mere knowledge of facts. For that reason my generation of orthopaedists accepted enthusiastically texts such as those by Vernon Luck,[58] Aegerter and Kirkpatrick,[1] McLean and Urist,[65] Salter,[81] and Rubin.[79] In dozens of sessions with such aid, those of my generation felt our way through poorly charted territories, using as foils the agile inquiring minds of such as Drs. R. Menke, P. MacFarland, H. Schoene, L. VanHerpe, H. Takahashi, E. Sedlin, C. Klasinski, P. Lehmuller, D. Carlson, and J. Lynch (who probably now play and enjoy similar roles with their own residents).

Be it known then, if knowledge consists of a vast catalog of facts, understanding consists of the very much simpler and far smaller but immensely more valuable and versatile catalog of the principles of action that cause natural things to dance their dance. In a manner of speaking, understanding represents the objectives and principles of the choreography, and if one knows them he need not memorize the enormous number of separate steps and maneuvers in nature's dance routine, for with the aid of the former and with little effort he can deduce the latter on the spot and as he needs them.

We will try to identify and use such principles here.

To do so efficiently we need a few special ideas and some terms having clearly understood meanings, and this first chapter will define and describe them, thereby setting the stage for what follows.

At the outset, plant this idea in your mind: the relatively simple but important physiological activities characteristic of the skeleton derive from a very simple kind of "alphabet" with which nature created a biological "language" which records the "stories" of our skeletons. These stories include its *evolution* (i.e. phylogeny), *ontogeny* (i.e. embryology), *growth*, and finally its *diseases* (i.e. pathology). In a very valid, even if abstract, sense, one cannot really understand these stories (quite a different matter from describing or memorizing them) unless he knows and understands the usage nature made of the alphabet in recording them and the structure of the language she built out of that alphabet. The natural alphabet, in common with most alphabets invented by man, has relatively few and quite simple letters which assemble in various ways to construct biologically meaningful words, sentences, and paragraphs of increasing complexity and—take special note—of progressively evolving purpose, all of which form the essence of the "messages" contained in the language built of the skeletal alphabet. We will return later to this rather basic and intriguing way of organizing our thoughts about the skeleton.

On another tack now, to most physicians the term "systems analysis" sounds impressively erudite as it rolls off the tongue, perhaps only because it conveys no crisp and clear idea to them. The point of view and the strategy of analysing problems signified by that term can potentiate very greatly one's ability to systematize, retain, and use the burgeoning knowledge that floods all fields of medicine. To give that term some practical solidity then, let us for our own present needs, first define a system, then a systems analysis, and then describe some systems properties that will prove highly relevant to later chapters and volumes.

SYSTEMS CONCEPTS

Definition of a System

Since we discuss human physiology and not cybernetics, let a system stand here for a complex functional entity such as a man or an automobile (for functional read *behavioral, purposeful, endowed with the capability of performing purposeful action*). The outward actions of such entities arise from separate internal parts which interact with themselves and with our outside environment (for separate internal parts read such things as *functional modules, subsystems, organs, tissues, anatomical structures*). Norbert Wiener,[101] Ashby,[8] and Apter and Wolpert[3] provide more general definitions for any who might want them and who can wade through the math.

Whether one calls something a *system* unto itself, a *subsystem* of a larger entity, or a *supersystem* composed itself of many subentities depends solely on his point of view and purpose at the moment. Thus, to my dad, a general practitioner in his latter days, one man usually constituted a complete system; yet, to a sociologist he represents the simplest atomistic subsubsubsystem or unit building block of the highly complex and organized entity he names society. For our present needs the whole skeleton will represent a system and the whole man will form a supersystem.

Functions

In the human body, and speaking in functional rather than anatomical terms, various subsystems exist for one great and general reason or purpose: to provide particular and specifiable *functions* to the remainder of the body, which includes other separable physiological subsystems as well as the intact organism itself. Accordingly, throughout this text the term "function" will signify some particular and necessary contribution made by one specifiable (and usually internal) subsystem to the intact body.

Disease

Then, it follows that a malfunction in any important subsystem causes a *disease* of the intact organism. Note that, as for the case of subsystem, system, and supersystem definitions, the terms "function" and "malfunction" also depend upon the focus of one's interest at the moment. As examples, syndactyly forms a normal characteristic of a duck, but we consider it a disease in man, while the low skeletal mass/body-mass ratio of a perfectly healthy porpoise characterizes the human disease, osteoporosis.

Having provided a brief "feel" for what the term "system" signifies, now let us try to do the same for the term "systems analysis."

Systems Analyses

Implied in the above remarks were the following particular ideas: A system represents a complex *behavioral* entity composed of subsystems which *interact* with each other; the important modes of its behavior consist of those having *purpose;* and disease implies abnormal behavior or aborted purpose or *malfunction* of one or more internal subsystems. Therefore, function and malfunction imply underlying *cause-effect* interactions. Finally, that biological systems also demonstrate considerable *organization* of their internal functions implies internal *cause-effect chains* that connect with varying degrees of complexity the behavioral characteristics of intact organisms to their ultimate macromolecular-level basis. Figure 1.01 diagrams the structural essence of the cause-effect chains found in bone as an organ (but ignores its lymphatic, vascular, and nerve supply).

In large part, this and the next two volumes in this series concentrate upon identifying and characterizing a few of the major cause-effect chains involved in the skeletal systems, chains which bridge the interval between the cell and the entire skeleton.

Keep this in mind, then: Normal bodily function as well as disease always represent the externally obvious results of *sequentially interconnected, internal, cause-effect chains* leading down eventu-

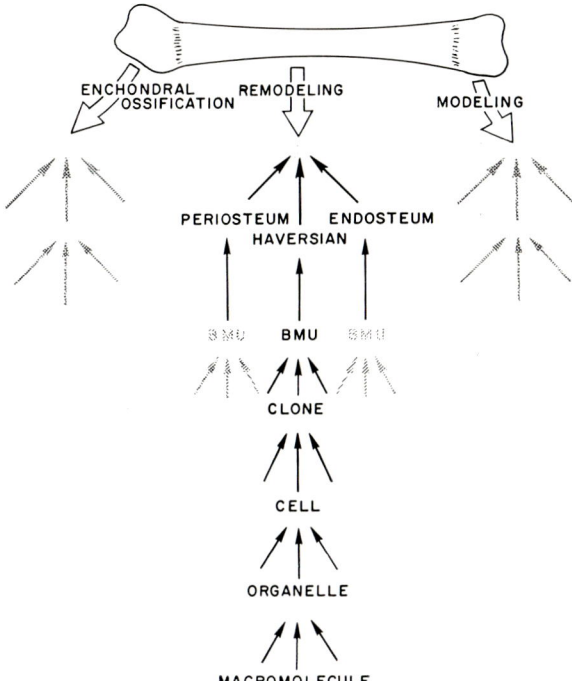

Figure 1.01. This diagrams or maps in brief form some of the currently identified number of levels of organization in the skeleton, the basis for their identification lying partly on functional and partly on morphological knowledge. A more comprehensive map will appear in Chapter X; you might inspect its figures briefly before going on, for that will give you some idea of where we will go. An important point shown by this scheme is that a very large number of molecular-level interactions at the bottom can participate, via upward-tending but converging chains of increasingly higher-order functions, in determining the properties and behavior of the intact organ. In this drawing, the three arrows converging from below on each level signify the fact that a variety of lower-level building blocks usually *associate* to create entirely new functional units at the next higher level.

ally and usually to the macromolecular level. We shall find later that this chain-like property has some intriguing spin-off effects on physiological behavior.

Then, to make clinical sense, any analysis of (as an example) endochondral bone formation must describe in cause-effect contexts the behavioral chains which relate it to normal growth and function, to aging, and to disease. Take special note here: *to do so one must know the particular functions that system exists to provide.* Analysing behavior as it relates to function and purpose constitutes part of what the term "systems analysis" means.

For that reason the systems analyses appearing herein simply tie the major functional, behavioral, and cause-effect features of a system together into a kind of dynamic, coordinated, and purposeful *gestalt* which relates healthy and pathological function and purpose to structure and composition. While picking something out and stating that our Maker made of it a function rather than a trivial phenomenon poses great risk of personal error (I certainly have no claim to any direct pipeline to His thinking), we must try to do exactly that in order to make better and more logical sense of matters. So I will try, and hope that others may identify and correct (and forgive) any errors that arise in the doing.

The Meaning and Relationship of Functions in the Economy of Intact Organisms

The term "function" appeared several times above as though it conveyed self-evident meaning. Consider for a moment the relationships between a man and his kidney, the latter and its nephrons, and the man and his nephrons. It sounds like hair-splitting, but not so.

One need hardly explain to this audience why the functions of the kidney as an organ depend on the underlying functions of nephrons. As perusal of Best and Taylor taught many of us, glomerular filtration, tubular reabsorption and secretion, and adjusting acid-base imbalances all represent functions supplied to the kidney as an organ by the summed-up behavior of numerous individual nephrons. Now, the kidney depends absolutely upon its nephrons to perform its specific functions and for its very existence as an entity with characteristic functional properties. Consequently, one might succumb to the temptation to assume that the man also depends absolutely upon his nephrons (i.e. no live nephrons—no live man, because no live nephrons—no live kidney).

With respect to the man, the functions supplied directly to him by his kidney as an organ form *first-order functions;* those supplied first and directly by nephrons to his kidney and then as an integrated and coordinated sum to the man form *second-order functions*. If one proceeds further downwards he can perceive third, fourth, and even higher-order functions. We can write this as a brief word equation, thus:

EQUATION 1

Intact man ⇌ Kidney ⇌ Nephrons ⇌ Cells

In this equation the arrows signify the interaction which represents the functions. In those terms, then, and by definition, removal of a first-order function causes a disease. Consequently, when first-order renal functions to the whole man (not the same thing as the renal organ) disappear, he indeed dies. It follows that were nephrons essential to human life, removing them would also kill a man.

By now you sense the argument's direction. We can and do remove kidneys and still maintain life by repeated dialysis. Dialysis does not replace even one-tenth of one per cent of the properties of the missing organs, but it does duplicate those very few and special properties of interaction which represent their *functions*.

Functions in biological organisms usually array in a kind of cascade or avalanche structure, of which we will say more in subsequent chapters.

As one example, the genes encoding the ability to synthesize collagen have exactly and only that as their first-order functional purpose. That purpose relates in no way predictable *a priori* to several organ level skeletal purposes (which that substance participates in realizing), such as allowing us to move about in our environment, to contain fluid under pressure, or to protect the skin from mechanical disruption.

As shown in Figure 1.02, one finds a close parallelism between the structural cascade of biological form and the functional cascade just mentioned. Only the naive would expect that structure always makes self-evident the function it provides. In point of fact, functions are often passing subtle.

10   *The Physiology of Cartilaginous, Fibrous, and Bony Tissue*

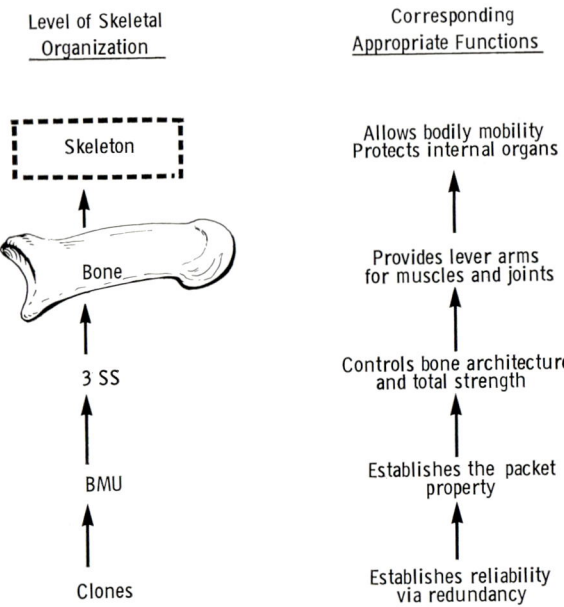

Figure 1.02. On the left, a diagrammatic representation of the evolution of biological organization within some particular organ. On the right, some of the purposes (first-order functions) supplied by a given level to the next higher one. Note that the purposes for which the organ may exist in the intact body may bear little direct relation to the functions provided by its cells; and in this particular scheme, organ level functions constitute fourth-order functions of individual cells. We will make the point later—and several times—that many functionally useful properties of organs are peculiar to the *pattern* in which various types of cells assemble or associate and have no representation in the properties of the individual cells in the patterns. Thus, a bone is strong in compression but none of its cells are; the heart pumps blood, although none of its muscle cells can do so individually.

Henceforth, use of the word "function" will accompany some statement or implication of the context in which it serves.

Elements of Control System Theory and Terminolgy

Increasingly, physicians encounter terms such as "feedback," "transducer," "negative feedback," and related words. Our residents tend to have very vague ideas of what these terms represent, although the concepts they designate provide powerful mental tools for augmenting our comprehension of, and ability to perceive, disease, as well as our therapeutic flexibility. Since many parts of these volumes deal with physiological behavior which one can understand and manipulate best in terms of control system concepts, this section will "translate" them from technical jargon into a form readily useable by an orthopaedic surgeon or his resident.

Let us begin by defining a control system (see Ashby[8]).

Control System

This designates any arrangement for controlling the behavior of any dynamic system, whether the latter represents a mechanical machine, a chemical process, an electronic amplification of sound, an economic system, a society, a man, or his skeleton. To manage the problem of conceptualizing the matter, control-system theory considers all such systems to have two "ends" or *interfaces* through which they interact with the world beyond them, even though an obvious physical or mechanical part may not actually correspond to those interfaces. The concept, after all, serves operational needs, not necessarily morphological ones. At one interface, the *output,* appears that behavior (i.e. the purposeful effects exerted on the world outside of it) which the control system exists to control; at the other, the *input,* appear all of those factors that help to control the system's responses to changes at the output, and so which manipulate the behavior of the system under control. Let us next crystallize further the ideas of behavior, input, and output.

Behavior

In our real world this designates *change in relation to time* (mathematicians can construct systems in which change occurs in relation to things other than time, but these need not concern us here). Note that you as an outside observer may see, as a consequence of such behavior, an obvious *active change* such as the take-off of a jet aircraft, or *no change,* as in the fixed relationship between the lens and its retaining cell in a microscope eyepiece. In the latter case, lack of appreciable change in the rela-

12 *The Physiology of Cartilaginous, Fibrous, and Bony Tissue*

tionship of the two parts over time represents exactly the desired result of control over the system's mechanical behavior, just as much as the behavior of the jet in response to the pilot's manipulation of its controls represents the exactly desired mechanical result. Think for a moment: were it otherwise, how useful would you find a microscope whose lenses changed alignment with the slightest jar or motion?

A control system acts to control the behavior of some system. This implies a further property: *it controls a particular form of behavior.* For example, the parathyroid gland exists to aid in controlling the level of ionized calcium in the serum; governments exist to control the behavior of human as well as of corporate and other purely legal beings; typewriter keys exist to control the motions of the type face.

A most important subclass of control systems depends for proper operation upon feedback, so let us turn to that next.

Feedback

This signifies in some way relaying or *feeding* information about the *output* behavior of some system *back* to its *input* facilities, with the control-oriented purpose of "informing" the latter of the behavior of the former. It therefore implies some means of sensing the behavior at the output (the *output sensor*), some means of relaying that information back to the input (i.e. the *feedback loop*), and some means of receiving the information transmitted thereby (the *input sensor*). Figure 1.03 diagrams a conventional general scheme for a feedback control system.

Such feedback of information implies some associated *purpose*, and in fact two important categories of such purposes do exist, diametrically opposite in their intended effects on the system's behavior. We acknowledge that circumstance when we speak of *positive feedback, negative feedback,* and/or the respective feedback *modes* of control.

Positive Feedback Mode

In this arrangement, a change at the output of the system becomes detected, travels back to the input along some kind of feed-

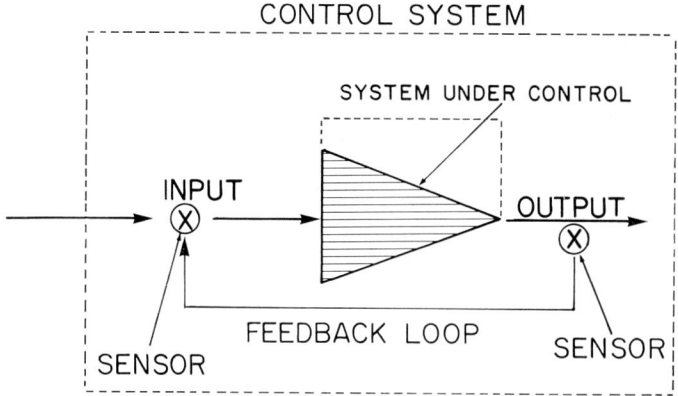

Figure 1.03. This diagrams the essential sequences and information-processing operations in a control system. Note that in an operational view the control apparatus exists in addition to or outside of the system under control. In natural systems, however, all parts usually come ingeniously and compactly packaged and defy recognition unless one approaches them with the special kind of insight we try to acquire here. Any introductory text about operational amplifiers and analog computers will expand considerably on this basic idea.

back loop, and there *acts to exaggerate the original output change.* This generates further feedback to the input, which further exaggerates the change, and so on. Common language terms such behavior a vicious cycle, an explosion, or a runaway type of behavior. When they occur very quickly we commonly and readily recognize them as explosions (example: a firecracker, which explodes in less than .005 second), but if they evolve over very long periods of time relative to our own perception of time, such as the astronomical evolution of galactic systems or the physiological evolution of our own brain, it may become quite difficult to recognize the essential control system mode characteristic; they tend at first glance to resemble equilibrium situations.

Particular examples of positive feedback systems in action will help to communicate further the essential idea.

1. *Explosion of Gunpowder:* In a cartridge, as the handloading authority Philip Sharpe noted, the particular controlled parameter consists of pressure. The flash of the primer ignites some of the

powder grains which convert to the much more voluminous gaseous state. Due to the small space in the cartridge case, the pressure rises and so does the temperature. This causes more powder grains to ignite, which further raises pressure and temperature, which ignites more powder grains, and so on. This powder would take several whole seconds to burn were it spilled loose on a table top and ignited with a match; because of the positive feedback just described, it burns within a very few thousandths of a second when confined within the cartridge case, and as a result it generates pressures measured in tons per square inch. That pressure (not temperature) represents the controlled parameter in this system, for exactly that propels the bullet out of the barrel of the gun and represents the *purpose* of the powder-barrel-bullet system. In this system the temperature simply represents a feedback mechanism or loop.

2. *Population Explosions:* These occupy a vastly longer time scale, yet otherwise have exactly the same operational control system elements. Accordingly, some 150,000 years ago fewer than a million men lived in the whole world. Then, progressively improving mastery over environment and disease increased individual survival time and so the number of people of reproductive age; that led to more children and better control of environmental and endogenous adversities, which led to more people, who produced more children, and so on. This particular "explosion," now at the stage of three billion or so souls, should reach some kind of conclusion within the next 100 years. Conceivably, like a culture of bacteria, we could exhaust our food-producing capacity (with the aid of environmental pollution) and thereby become extinct. More likely, to my mind, we will learn to handle these problems as (according to historians such as Gibbons) the Romans learned to handle, at least in the immediate sense, their garbage and sewage disposal problems some 2000 years ago, and as we have learned to control bacterial disease within the past century. To my mind, a far more ominous threat to our collective survival looms, like thunderheads on the horizon, in another direction entirely: into the hands of a species capable of cooperative malice, bias, bigotry, hate, violence, and true vicious-

ness, men such as Einstein, Bohr, and Planck unlocked and placed some of the destructive as well as constructive capacities residing within atoms and radiant energy. Ominous, because we demonstrate far less wisdom in controlling man than we do in controlling matter. The risk here lies not in the properties of matter and energy but rather to what use we ourselves shall put them.

3. *Septicemia:* Here bacteria multiply in the blood faster than the body's defenses can subdue them; more bacteria divide to produce more daughter duplicates which in turn divide, and so on, until the very mass of their chemical excreta fatally poisons the patient.

Negative Feedback Mode

Most physiological control mechanisms function in this mode, and so most readers have seen this term more often than its antonym. In this arrangement the control system confines or restrains some parameter within limits compatible with optimum health and functional potential. That parameter might constitute the concentration of an inorganic ion or a hormone molecule in the blood, the shape of a bone relative to the mechanical loads it carries, or the process of cell division as it relates to growth and maintenance-related bodily activities. It works as follows:

The sensor mechanism *monitoring* the output of the system generates an appropriate signal from any error in that output and relays it back to the input along the feedback loop. At the input that signal then causes the control mechanism to change the system's behavior *in that particular way which acts to reduce the error.* Thus, two important behavioral characteristics of (and consequently clues to the presence of) any negative feedback control arrangement are the following:

1. The controlled parameter varies only within certain limits, and should it depart from them some *active* process returns it within those limits.

2. A *time lag* always separates the development of an error and its subsequent correction.

It may help to clarify this idea by describing it as another simple word equation, thus:

EQUATION 2

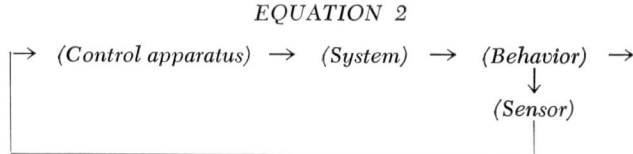

Examples of negative feedback system would include:

3. *Parathyroid Control of Hypocalcemia:* F. C. McLean found long ago that when the level of ionized calcium in the arterial blood entering the parathyroid glands falls, it causes the gland to increase its secretion of parathormone (PTH).[65] PTH acts on a variety of interfaces between the blood and the rest of the body (i.e. bone, kidney, gut) *in such a way as to raise the seruim calcium.* That rise returns the ionized calcium in the blood to normal, whereupon the stimulus that had turned the glands "on" disappears and so they now turn "off." Since the system actually functions with gradations of response rather than in the all-or-none fashion just used for clear communication, and since it exhibits a very large capacity to correct errors, it maintains a fairly narrowly defined level of calcium ion concentration even in the presence of large challenges.

We will mention later some physiological and cybernetic equivalents of Sherlock Holmes' "dog that did not bark." This signifies that when something consistently does not happen in a dynamic system whose nature provides plenty of opportunity for it to do so, the underlying reason almost always consists of a negative feedback control system which *actively controls and constrains* the parameter in question. Thus, and as an example, the fact that in healthy people the larger of two tendons *invariably* belongs to the muscle with the greater contractile force (a property I invoked in Volume I to determine in the operating room which peroneal muscle had the greatest contractile force and therefore which should be transferred to provide the greatest corrective force) constitutes a physiological dog that did not bark, for otherwise as they enlarge far more than a hundredfold between embryonic life and the age of skeletal maturity (and were their growths in diameter controlled independently of their muscles' contractile force), many instances should arise—due to random biologic variation—of mismatches between muscle force and tendon strength.

Similarly with the alignment of the knee, ankle, elbow and interphalangeal joints, and the normal gross anatomical curves of bones such as the clavicle, ribs, radius and femur.

THE SCOPE

This text concerns the skeleton, which contains primarily cartilaginous, bony, and fibrous tissues. Five factors will help to understand and to place the textual material in perspective, relative to what you know already about physiology. These factors include (a) the level of organization gap, (b) a basis for defining a functional entity or uniqueness, (c) the problem of our terminology, (d) the problem of one's analytical strategy, and (e) the three faces of disease.

Level of Organization Gap

In the medical research, studies of the cell as an entity and level of biological organization, on the one hand, and of the skeleton as an entity and level of organization, on the other, have taught us much of interest and importance and will continue to do so in the foreseeable future. However, a very large gap exists in our contemporary understanding (which is more than knowledge) of what happens between these two levels, although studies published within the last decade uncover features in that region of crucial importance to any realistic understanding of the functions of the body's component cells (Jee et al,[51] Weiss,[100] Polanyi,[71] Villanueva and Frost[98]). These studies justify the following categorical statement:

One cannot understand bodily function solely in terms of cellular function.

The foregoing statement holds true in spite of the obvious reality that in the collective sense cells lie at the bottom of all skeletal development, growth, and function. To record a relevant but perhaps more obvious analogy, no more could one understand an automobile wheel's function and design solely in terms of the properties of its component atoms. Its function makes sense *only when related to the rest of the car;* its design makes sense *only in relation to its function.* This remains as true of skeletons as of wheels.

These texts occupy (and perhaps preoccupy) themselves in various ways with this less studied "in-between region" of skeletal organization, including its relation to skeletal functions and diseases of clinical concern. Do not minimize the importance of this region: it holds major answers to a variety of eye-catching problems with which orthopaedists deal, or over which we ponder when the state of our art makes us unable to deal effectively with them. Representative problems would include organ and limb regeneration (Becker,[11] Bassett *et al*[12]); fracture and nerve repair (Urist *et al*[97]); controlling the growth process to correct congenital anatomical deficiencies; and developing routinely successful internal, inanimate prostheses for bones, joints, tendons, and muscles until such time as we can make the body regenerate its own new and living replacements. Once daydreams, these things have now become rather clearly possible in principle, removed from us only by our own present lack of understanding. So, while some new facts may appear in these pages, most of them relate a few things possibly new to most readers to far more numerous and older facts and within a utilitarian and clinically oriented context.

A Basis for Recognizing Functional Subsystems

Ultimately, what justifies distinguishing as separate functional entities any of the various cellular systems in our bodies? Or to put it another way, how do we know in distinguishing fibrous bone from lamellar bone that we sort out meaningful facts and do not split hairs in a trivial way?

I propose here that the ultimate (and purely operational) justification for such distinctions represents the capacity of such a singled-out system to develop one or more diseases peculiar to itself—i.e. which do not inherently involve malfunctions of other cellular systems. Deceptively simple, this strategic axiom really has considerable analytical depth. All distinctions made in this text between different cellular systems or between different cellularly-based behavioral entities will lie on such a base. Note that besides being subject to its own peculiar diseases any such system also can participate in others which do affect other cellular systems.

Our knowledge of molecular biology provides a ready explanation for such behavior. To illustrate, a coding error of congenital origin in that part of the cell's DNA that specifies the amino acid sequences in collagen should cause disease only in tissues to which collagen provides some necessary function; on that basis one could predict accurately the identity of such tissues (cartilage, dermis, fascia, tendon, dentine, bone). A coding error in an enzyme necessary for Krebs cycle function would affect all cells and most severely those that metabolize the fastest, for ultimately the life of all of our cells depends upon carbohydrate-derived energy supplied by the Krebs cycle.

> *Note:* The existence of a disease which causes a malfunction peculiar to one particular cellular system (of any degree of complexity) indicates this, among other things: *one or more regulatory factors unique to that system exist.* Therefore, and until one understands all physiology sufficiently exhaustively to account for such pecularities precisely and accurately, it behooves us to consider cellular systems manifesting diseases peculiar to themselves as functional entities. While not a wholly conventional view, nevertheless, considerable and convincing justification exists for such an approach.

Terminology

This field has a confused and inconsistent terminology, and even Dorland's latest medical dictionary can help a student little here. The terminology arose to serve communication needs and a level of understanding extant more than a generation ago; since then a true revolution has occurred in our grasp of skeletal physiology and the way in which we look at it, partly by way of infusions of new insight from multiple other areas of science and technology. Consequently, the older terminology not only communicates increasingly ineffectively; on occasion it actually misleads.

In part, this problem requires defining terms as we use them and collecting those definitions in a glossary at the end of the book. In part and as appropriate, I will describe specific inadequacies of the older terminology, not to inflate myself by deflating something else but so that the reader can understand better the usage of such terms found in older texts or in modern research reported in older language and concepts.

Strategy

Working out the relationships described herein followed a systems analysis, performed in somewhat spotty fashion in that the analytical activity stretched with gradually increasing precision and acuity over 25 years of my medical career. It pursued a special strategy which proved very efficient and which talented and honored engineers and research people outside of medicine find almost self-evident and axiomatic* (and thus not seeming to need any defense), but which, at least in my own experience, people in medicine tend to find peculiarly unsettling. This strategy will be described at the end of this volume.

The Three Faces of Disease

Figure 1.04 introduces what I feel comprises a useful and important if simple concept. Specifically, *all* biological phenomena depend ultimately upon cellular proliferation and differentiation, and one whole class of diseases arises primarily as errors in the normal patterns of those activities. A second far better known and studied but subsidiary class I term "biochemical disease," signifying abnormal patterns of biochemical activities within already existing populations of differentiated cells. A third very poorly known and equally subsidiary class consists of those situations in which for one or another reason the orientation in space

---

*At the Bone Workshop at Sun Valley, Idaho, July, 1971, sponsored by the NIDR and the University of Utah School of Medicine, I had the opportunity to listen to Drs. Hector Deluca and David Howell describe (totally unaware of the direction and nature of my interest) how, in their own research, which in my opinion is truly outstanding, they had unwittingly followed exactly that strategy. My experience has been that most unusually effective scientists have the inborn knack of doing that.

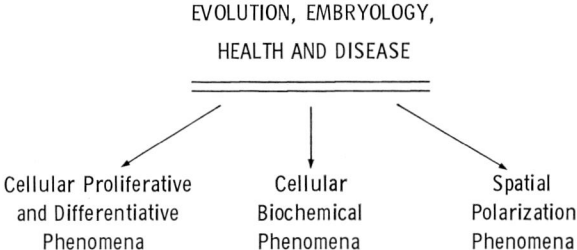

Figure 1.04. The three "faces" of disease, as well as of its underlying determinants. These faces represent distinctive classes of biological phenomena whose aberrations produce equally distinctive classes of diseases. Medicine to date has preoccupied itself with biochemical aspects of disease as it arises in already existing populations of differentiated cells. Pharmacology and anesthesiology belong peculiarly and nearly exclusively to it. Disproportionately much less attention has been given to diseases arising from defective proliferation and differentiation (most congenital anomalies lie in this class), and almost none to spatial polarization phenomena, although an orthopaedist encounters the latter daily in the clinic and operating room. The lack of extant literature and expertise dealing with these other two faces of disease does not reflect accurately any low importance in the scale of things; rather, it reflects a rather slow and off-balance awakening to their real and great importance on our part.

of various cellular activities becomes disturbed. Usually in any physiological system we find all three of these aspects combined and intimately interwoven, a matter which undoubtedly has contributed to our tardy recognition of each as a functional and *clinically important* entity unto itself.

This volume deals much more with the first and third categories, not because of any intent to belittle the second but rather in an effort to improve the contemporary imbalance among them, an effort necessitated by the aforesaid neglect of the other two. This concept of disease deserves some amplification to make it more useful to you, and the concluding chapters of a later volume will do just that.

QUESTIONS

1. Define a system. List examples in medicine, society, and astronomical physics.

2. Define a function; define a disease.
3. How do first-order functions differ from second and higher-order ones?
4. List some examples of negative feedback as it operates in human physiology; in economic theory; in arms races.
5. Describe at least one useful way to distinguish between different cellular systems.

Chapter II

The Basic Functional Plan of the Skeleton

Organizationally, the skeleton represents a "paragraph" built with an "alphabet" of letters comprising its simple tissues and the simple and few activities and functions each letter provides and subserves. By combining letters into separate "words" and "sentences," the paragraph representing the intact skeleton arises. In this building process, structure always associates with behavior and functional purpose, and all evolve and transform as one ascends the organizational ladder. Thus, the immediate purposes of an intact bone bear little obvious parallel with the immediate purposes of the cells that made it.

INTRODUCTION

As mentioned previously, the skeletal system exhibits organization of its structure and of the composition of the matter which composes it. Of even more importance its functions also exhibit organization, and a parallelism characterizes its physical properties and its physiological functions. As a problem unto itself, many schemes and approaches exist which try to make the biological organization of the skeleton logical and lucid; see, as examples Lacroix,[55] Putschar,[72] and Johnson[53] (or J. Trueta's relatively recent book). Let us here sketch in a preliminary and skeletal way some of the main features of this organization according to a scheme of my own, to help later in plugging numerous details into their proper place in the overall picture. This "plugging" process assumes great importance in understanding things but often obtains short shrift in our literature. I refer interested readers to a few stellar examples of effective plugging (Jacob and Monod,[49] Polanyi,[71] Jee et al,[51] Epker,[27] Arnold,[4,5] Heaney,[47] Harris and Heaney,[46] Johnson,[53] Hall,[44] Young[104]). Let us do this through the alphabet analogy, in which each letter and word associates with corresponding structures and purposes. Just as man uses simple binary (i.e. "yes or no" or "zero and one") bits to construct powerful and versatile computers which can calculate, predict, write music, and translate books, so nature used these simple elements to evolve and construct the neuromusculoskeletal system with all of its complexity, engineering exactness, and variety. Because each letter and higher construct in this language has abstract, morphological, chemical, behavioral, and purposeful properties or aspects associated with it, let us identify some of them next to provide some idea of how they build, one upon the other, and how the various aspects evolve in parallel to each other.

The Abstract Sense

The skeleton's basic "alphabet" contains only a few "letters" (we deal with five here) which can assemble in various but again in few ways to form a variety of different "words"; the latter assemble into sentences and then paragraphs, and so on.

The Structural Sense

Each of those five letters represents a *simple tissue*. Combining these tissues in various ways (we observe only nine such ways in human skeletal physiology) builds more complex and highly organized "words" termed "complex tissues." Both simple and complex tissues combine in a few particular ways to build "sentences" or *organs;* the assemblage of all of its essential organs into their natural relationships constitutes a "paragraph" called the *skeleton,* a supersystem relative to a single bone.

In the Sense of Behavior

Each letter signifies two things: the ability to *make* the tissue involved and later to *remove* it. By combining various letters or simple tissues in controlled sequences, these simple modes of behavior can produce complex structures such as epiphyses, osteochondromas, diaphyses, and spongy bone. By combining those complexes in particular ways and sequences one produces organs.

In the Sense of Purpose

Each letter provides a few basic first-order purposes or functions which we describe shortly; by combining them into words

The Basic Functional Plan of the Skeleton

more highly evolved and complex (and even totally new), purposes become realized; by combining all into a paragraph, still higher purposes become realized. To provide an initial idea of what those paragraphs mean, Table 2.01 outlines from the purely structural viewpoint the progression in skeletal organization, from the most elementary on the left to the most highly organized and complex on the right.

Now let us retrace several parts of that path in slightly greater detail.

TABLE 2.01
ASCENDING SKELETAL ORGANIZATION

Simple Tissues →	Complex Tissues →	Organ →	Superorgan
Fibrous tissue	Articular cartilage	Femur	The intact skeleton
Fibrous bone	Epiphysis	Tibia	+ Voluntary muscle ↓
Lamellar bone	Epiphyseal plate	Parietal bone	The musculoskeletal system
Hyaline cartilage	Intervertebral disc	Anterior cruciate ligament	+ Nervous system ↓
Fibrocartilage	Spongiosa		The neuromusculoskeletal system
Others (marrow lymphatic vascular innervation)	Compacta	Interosseous membrane	
	Metaphysis	EPL tendon	
	Diaphysis	Tendo achillis	
Muscle tissue	Capsule	Hip joint	
	Ligament	Muscle (complete)	
	Tendon		
	Muscle belly		

This table lists specific examples of the purely structural progression of skeletal organization, beginning with "letters" in the left-hand column and progressing to whole paragraphs in the right-hand column. No attempt is made here to specify how many elements assemble, or in what order, to form the structures designated in the more right-hand columns. That task will be done later on and piece by piece.

THE SKELETAL ALPHABET
Skeletal Letters

In the anatomical or structural sense, and for our needs, five basic letters of the skeletal alphabet exist. They constitute what we will call the *simple tissues* of the skeletal system; *they provide the base for all skeletal growth, physiology, and disease,* and they include the following:

Hyaline cartilage.
Fibrocartilage.
Fibrous bone.
Lamellar bone.
Fibrous tissue.

Switching from the morphological to the behavioral sense now, those tissues or letters provide the following first-order activities:

Production and resorption of cartilage.
Production and resorption of fibrous bone and similarly of lamellar bone.
Production and removal of fibrous tissue.

Those functional activities subserve specific purposes, some of which Table 2.02 lists. We shall pretty much ignore here certain

TABLE 2.02
SIMPLE SKELETAL TISSUES

Structural Name	Behavorial Property Provided	Some Purposes Subserved
Hyaline cartilage	Production Resorption (after mineralization)	Creation *de novo* of new skeletal tissue; growth regulation by endocrine and biomechanical factors; joint lubrication and load-carrying needs; repair
Fibrocartilage	Production Resorption	Flexible pressure-carrying pads for distributing loads across joints
Fibrous bone	Production Resorption (after mineralization)	Creation *de novo* of new skeletal tissue; an essential intermediary in replacement activities; repair
Lamellar bone	Production Resorption (after mineralization)	To remain rigid under compression and shearing loads; to supply an electrolyte and buffer reservoir to the blood; to resist mechanical fatigue failure
Fibrous tissue	Production Resorption	To remain rigid under tension loads

The left column of this table identifies the skeleton's five chief *simple tissues*. The middle column names some of the behavioral activities with which they endow the body, while the right-hand column lists some of the major purposes subserved by the behavior characteristic of each tissue. These purposes represent functions supplied by these tissues to higher levels of organization in the skeletal system.

other simple tissues, such as the soft tissues in the bone marrow (although as Frame and Nixon point out,[30] they probably play a meaningful role in the overall scheme of the skeleton), the bone's innervation, and its vascular supply. That does not mean I hold them unimportant (quite the contrary); I do it to promote clarity and to minimize any confusion arising from presenting more detail than our minds can absorb readily. Figure 2.01 relates these tissues to the skeleton and also in a preliminary way to each other, diagrammatically.

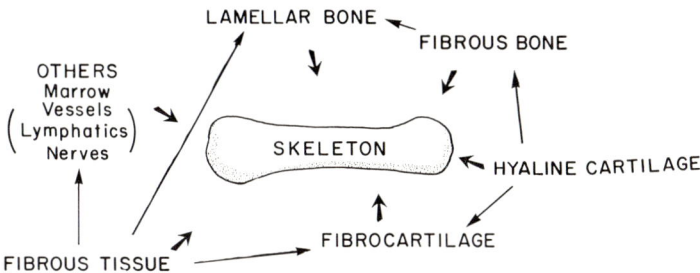

Figure 2.01. In the last analysis the intact skeleton represents the summated contributions of its simple tissues, which initially provided and then built further upon its embryological anlages. This diagram illustrates that fact and also a further point, not particularly emphasized in this part of the text, that some of these tissues interact with each other (first-order interactions) to form new complexes that in turn give rise to specific necessary higher-order contributions to the whole.

As indicated, the structural letters supply a few but very important basic physiological purposes or functions; they include the following specific ones:

1. *Hyaline cartilage* exhibits the important property that it can arise *de novo* where no rigid skeletal tissue existed before. Thereby, it provides the essential initial step of one of the only two basic mechanisms known in the entire animal kingdom for creating new bony tissue where none existed previously. To emphasize the importance of those two mechanisms, in growth and disease as well as during skeletal evolution, no examples of bony tissue arriving on any other paths than those two have ever been iden-

tified in any paleontological study of skeletal evolution (see Enlow[24, 25, 26] for further information on this), in any species of animal known to man anywhere on the face of the earth, nor in any disease known to medical or veterinary science.

Elastically deformable like bone, unlike it hyaline cartilage displays relatively high mechanical compliance in all directions (meaning it "gives" more easily in response to external mechanical forces applied to it from any direction); that promotes the uniform distribution of loads across joints, a useful property because nonuniform distribution can lead to so-called traumatic arthritis. Some of its chemical and physical properties play a vital role in its lubricity, which promotes its lasting service as a bearing material for all sliding joints.

The speed of its growth responds in characteristic ways to externally applied mechanical forces (the Heuter-Volkmann relation and my own correlaries to it, described in Ch. VI), thereby providing the mechanism that establishes the shapes of developing and growing joints. Its speed of growth also comes directly under the control of growth hormone (STH) so that all growing cartilaginous structures display a very high degree of overall coordination and parallelism.

2. *Fibrocartilage* apparently arises only where some kind of skeletal tissue existed previously (I am uncertain of this because we understand fibrocartilage much less than the hyaline variety and we know even less of elastic cartilage). It possesses anisotropic mechanical compliance, meaning that in response to mechanical compression and tension loads it "gives," and more readily in some directions than in others. This makes it *strong* so as to resist disruption, yet allows it to remain *flexible* so it can adapt to irregular underlying bony surfaces where it serves as a pad to distribute mechanical loads evenly across poorly fitting joint surfaces, as in the knee and the vertebral endplates. These properties minimize the danger of structural damage to underlying and much more pressure-sensitive tissues, damage which could arise if localized areas of overload developed.

3. *Fibrous bone* can also arise where no rigid skeletal tissue previously existed, and it thus provides the essential initial step

for the second known way of creating new bony tissue where none existed before. Relative to the skeleton's own natural time scale (for example, the period of time required for the growing human skeleton to mature), fibrous bone can arise quickly (typically within two weeks) and in voluminous amounts. In bulk it possesses less mechanical compliance than cartilage but more than lamellar bone, and it displays essentially isotropic compliance at the naked eyelevel of resolution, i.e. it has no effective gross-level "grain."

4. *Lamellar bone* can deposit only on preexisting bone, regardless of whether that consists of the fibrous or lamellar type. Thus, whenever you see lamellar bone in a microscopic section, its existence *proves* the previous initial act of either hyaline cartilage creation and/or fibrous bone formation. It also proves the existence of sufficient elapsed time for these transitions to occur, typically not less than three months. Information such as this can on occasion help to interpret bone pathology. Lamellar bone has a structural grain and high anisotropy of mechanical compliance, for like wood it displays much greater stiffness (and strength too) parallel to its grain than across it. If by some means one were to align this oriented strength parallel to the major mechanical loads carried by a bony part, this would make lamellar bone superior as a structural material to fibrous bone and to cartilage of either type. Similarly, forged pliers have greater strength than cast ones, because the forging process aligns the grain structure in such a way as to best sustain the forces to which one normally subjects a pair of pliers.

In point of fact, a very important biological mechanism does exist which aligns the grain of lamellar bone in exactly that manner. It receives detailed attention in the fourth volume of this series as the *flexure-drift relations* described therein, which can predict the specific architectural behavior of a bone in the operational sense with great clinical confidence.

5. *Fibrous tissue* exists to carry tension loads (i.e. to provide low compliance and high strength and stiffness in tension) but to deform readily under compression and shear loads. As we shall see when we discuss scar and mature fibrous tissue forma-

tion, a mechanism that aligned the grain of fibrous tissues parallel to the tension loads they typically carry would allow maximal mechanical efficiency with a minimum of material, while a separate mechanism that dealt out the total amount of collagen in proportion to need would match structural strength to functional demand. As for bone, such mechanisms do exist; they receive some attention in a later chapter of this volume as the stretch-hypertrophy rule.

Skeletal Words

In the Abstract Sense

To repeat: in life the preceding "letters" assemble into a dictionary of only nine oft-encountered basic "words"; again, the characteristic anatomical and compositional properties of each such word associate with typical activities and purposes.

In the Structural Sense

The words created by combining and/or modifying the five simple tissues represent *complex tissues*. Like the term "simple tissues" used previously, this term probably will be new to the reader because I coined it specifically for this book to fill a need. The term designates a structure either (a) built of two or more simple tissues (primary spongiosa, epiphysis, metaphysis); or (b) one simple tissue upon which additional structural order has been imposed beyond that which exists in the raw material of the tissue (trabeculae, cortex); or (c) some combination of both. Yet, a complex tissue does not exhibit sufficient organization or anatomical and functional separability from other constructs to justify calling it an organ. This of course forms an arbitrary choice, suitable here but under other possible circumstances and requirements needlessly restrictive and, so, dispensable.

Table 2.03 lists eight important complex skeletal tissues (the ninth simply representing an ordered combination of three of the eight*), and for each it also lists the characteristic histological

---

*See if you can identify the ninth by yourself.

composition, essential behavior, and some of the purposeful functions subserved by the tissue. We will consider some of this material in more detail later; here I want to provide some kind of bird's-eye overview of skeletal organization which, like a small-sized city map, allows one to locate particular parts and problems within the overall view or plan. By such means we obtain better perspective.

The table lists *articular cartilage, epiphyseal plate cartilage, epiphysis, primary spongiosa, secondary spongiosa, compacta, tendon insertion,* and *tendon* (as representative also of ligament and fascia) as the major skeletal complex tissues. In other words, where only five letters serve to create the basic building blocks for all skeletal growth, aging, disease, and evolutionary phenomena, only eight words made up with those letters have proved necessary to achieve the same ends. Consider articular cartilage, secondary spongiosa, and compacta briefly next, for doing so will help to explain why I distinguish them as complex tissues.

From the standpoint of their *organic chemical composition,* no significant difference exists between the simple tissue *hyaline cartilage,* and the complex tissue *articular cartilage* which after all is composed solely of hyaline cartilage. A difference in their inorganic composition does exist, for articular cartilage has at its bottom a mineralized layer, while the simple tissue need not. From the standpoint of the spatial order of its cellular and fibrillar components (collagen) at the light microscope level, considerable differences do exist between them, for the latter exhibits regular fibrillar order and alignment relative to the underlying (and thus subchondral) bone, as well as order in the way in which its proliferating and differentiated cells become arranged in space. This order participates in essential ways in its functions as articular cartilage. In fact, exactly that order endows the complex tissue with new properties *which the raw simple tissue alone does not possess.*

Similarly, *secondary spongiosa* simply consists of trabeculae (i.e. interlocking bars and/or plates) of lamellar bone, chemically indistinguishable from lamellar bone—the simple tissue of any source whatsoever within the growing or adult skeleton. Why,

TABLE 2.03

COMPLEX SKELETAL TISSUES ("WORDS")

Structural Name	Histological Composition (Simple Tissues)	Behavior Provided	Functions Subserved by Structure and Behavior
Articular cartilage	Hyaline cartilage with spatially oriented fibers and growth pattern	Enlargement in response to endocrine control; mechanical compliance; resists tangential shear; mechanical growth force-response characteristic	Lubrication (reduction of wear); mechanical shock dissipation; control of articular shape and alignment during growth
Epiphyseal cartilage	Hyaline cartilage with spatially oriented fibers and growth pattern	Spatially oriented enlargement	Longitudinal growth; mechanical support for epiphysis; limb alignment
Primary spongiosa	Calcified hyaline cartilage, fibrous bone	Production and replacement	Mechanical support for epiphyseal plate; permits replacement by trabecula of lamellar bone
Secondary spongiosa	Lamellar bone trabeculae	Production and replacement	Mechanical support for epiphyseal region; bone turnover; electrolyte-buffer reservoir
Compacta	Lamellar bone	Spatially oriented Production and replacement	Supplies rigidity in compression, tension, and shear. Allows mechanical needs to control shape and size; immune to fatigue; electrolyte-buffer reservoir
Tendon insertion	Tendon, cartilage, bone	Spatially oriented growth in response to endocrine and mechanical control	Supplies rigidity in tension and solid attachment to bone for transmitting tension forces to it

TABLE 2.03 (Continued)

Structural Name	Histological Composition (Simple Tissues)	Behavior Provided	Functions Subserved by Structure and Behavior
Tendon	Fibrous tissue with spatially oriented fibers	Production, replacement, and enlargement	Supplies rigidity and strength in tension to transmit tension loads from muscles to other structures
Epiphyseal complex	Calcified and uncalcified hayaline cartilage, fibrous bone, lamellar bone	Accumulation and replacement	Longitudinal growth; shaping articulations and aligning them

The common structural names of eight of the skeleton's *complex tissues* appear in the left-hand column. The second column lists either the simple tissues which compose them or the added degree of order that justifies designating them a more highly organized material than their chemical and histological components alone would suggest. The third column lists biological behavior typically associated with each complex tissue, while the last column lists some functions that behavior supplies to the intact skeleton. While proposing associations of specific purposes with specific structural features carries with it risk of error, such identifications are absolutely essential to rapid future progress in this whole field, and one must admire and applaud the efforts along these lines of authors such as E. Eisenberg, R. Heaney, J. S. Arnold, W. S. S. Jee, B. N. Epker, L. Mathews, L. C. Johnson, R. Talmage, L. Belanger, P. Meunier, Rutishauser, Vaes, R. Amprino, C. Anderson, C. Nordin, S. Garn, and many others.

therefore, distinguish them? Simple: the trabeculae in secondary spongiosa exhibit a particular type of architectural order and arrangement in tissue space which endows a mass of secondary spongiosa with new overall mechanical as well as physiological properties *which lamellar bone alone and as a raw material does not possess.*

Likewise for *compacta.*

Skeletal Sentences

In the Abstract Sense

Both simple "letters" and complex "words" combine in particular ways to produce "sentences," and these sentences also have structural, compositional, behavioral, and functional meanings, as follows.

Structurally Speaking

Inferring backwards now from functions rather than forwards solely from gross anatomical data (an important qualification and point of view), we can recognize at least three general types of bony organs: long bones with a definite diaphyseal or shaft-like region, which in the mechanical sense function primarily as columns, in that they sustain compression loads at either end (femur, vertebral, centrum, ilium); short, squat bones essentially composed of metaphysis and covered totally by cartilage (tarsal navicular, capitate, all sesamoids, including the patella); and flat bones, which normally carry no large compression loads (cranial vault).

Chemical Composition

Excepting their articulating surfaces, these bones have exactly similar properties in this sense, i.e. studies of their chemical composition cannot explain their differences in behavior and function. This holds true because lamellar bone, which possesses a defined chemical composition, provides the simple tissue used to build all of them.

Behavior

These organs exhibit several forms of behavior of major functional importance in the body's economy. These behavioral forms include overall enlargement during the growing period (i.e. *growth*); *replacement* of one tissue type (whether simple or complex) by another; patterned movement of their surfaces through tissue space in conformity to biomechanical needs (i.e. *modeling*); *mechanical rigidity and strength* under compression, tension, and shearing loads; and *exchange* of their chemical building stuffs with the blood.

Function

From this standpoint these organs subserve the needs of *creation;* of *growth;* of adapting both their ultimate sizes and their architecture to the requirements of biomechanical factors associated with gravity, muscle forces, and joint function; of allowing *motion* of one bone relative to others; of *aligning* and *stabilizing* the various bones of a limb; and of providing to the blood a large *reservoir* of electrolyte and acid base. Its investing cells also endow a bone with practical *immunity to mechanical fatigue failure*, with the capacity to *repair* injury, and with the ability to *defend* itself from bacteriological, chemical, thermal, neoplastic, and physical threats.

Table 2.04 lists some of these properties. The next few paragraphs expound briefly on the organ-level functional roles just listed. Before touching on them keep this thought in mind: *all* of them represent activities provided solely by assembling in various but well-defined ways the basic structural and behavioral properties of the five letters of this language, the simple skeletal tissues.

1. *Creation* herein means creating a new skeletal organ where only soft, nonskeletal tissue existed previously. Ultimately, only three cellularly based processes (i.e. functional letters) endow the normal body with this creative capability, to wit: *bone formation in membrane, chondrogenesis,* and *fibrogenesis.* Such crea-

36 *The Physiology of Cartilaginous, Fibrous, and Bony Tissue*

TABLE 2.04
BONY ORGANS

Structural Names	Histological Composition	Typical Behavior	Functions Subserved
Long hollow columnar bone (femur, ilium, mandible, rib)	Lamellar bone (trabecular and compact); hyaline cartilage (articular, tendon insertion, ligament insertion), marrow tissue	Rigid and strong in compression, shear, flexure, and torque: moves at articulations; turnover; blood-bone exchange; hematopoiesis	Carries muscular and gravitic loads, provides mechanical leverage to muscles, contains hematopoietic activity, exchanges electrolytes and buffer with blood, resists mechanical fatigue, allows mechanically controlled motion relative to other bones; growth and modeling
Long solid columnar bone (ear ossicles)	Compact lamellar bone only; hyaline cartilage (joints and tendon insertions)	As above except hematopoiesis	Carries compression loads generated by tympanic membrane, resists mechanical fatigue; growth and modeling
Short trabecular bone (navicular, patella)	Lamellar bone (trabecular and compact); hyaline cartilage; fibrocartilage, marrow tissue	Rigid and strong in compression and tension; hematopoiesis	Carries mechanical loads, contains hematopoietic activity, exchanges electrolytes and buffer with the blood, resists mechanical fatigue; growth and modeling
Flat bone (Parietal, frontal)	Lamellar bone (compacta and diploë), marrow tissue	Rigid in compression, tension, and shear; blood-bone exchange; hematopoiesis	Protects brain from impact, exchanges electrolyte and buffer with the blood, hematopoiesis, growth and modeling

The left column lists four functional and biomechanical types of bones, a scheme differing in some respects from the classical and purely anatomical ones that appear in anatomy textbooks. The second column lists the tissue elements that compose them, the third some obvious behavioral activities, and the last some obvious functions subserved by the organs. Note that at skeletal maturity the functions of growth and modeling (the latter serving in the sense of sculpting) become inactive and so would not participate in giving rise to skeletal diseases acquired during adult life.

The Basic Functional Plan of the Skeleton 37

tion occurs first and normally in the developing embryo; if it occurs subsequently it represents a consequence of repair or defense, or of the formation of a benign neoplasm (osteoma, myositis ossificans, enchondroma, osteochondroma or exostosis, fibroma, or a hamartoma) or of a malignant one (osteosarcoma, chondrosarcoma, fibrosarcoma).

Defective creative activities lead to missing members or parts of members and to supernumerary parts, both seen most commonly in a large variety of congenital deformities.

2. *Growth* at the organ level designates those activities which act to enlarge the size and mass of a bone from the fetal size to that of the mature adult. It involves separate activities for producing *growth in length,* and *growth in diameter,* and these activities include creation as just defined and replacement as next defined, all following an orderly and predictable pattern. Each of these two growth processes follows its own "rules" as far as responding to systemic regulation and biomechanical needs are concerned.

Defective longitudinal growth leads to various forms of generalized and localized dwarfism in the case of retardations, and to gigantism in the case of accelerations.

3. *Replacement* represents the ability first to remove an earlier produced tissue and then to deposit in its place another type of tissue (whether simple or complex). While certainly well known—without it the mammalian skeleton simply cannot arise—replacement activity has not previously received a proper identifying term.

Yet, the complicated series of replacement steps involved in producing any complete and mature mammalian skeleton probably exist in part because the lamellar bone which composes it cannot arise *de novo,* meaning in the absence of any kind of preexisting bone.

Defective replacement activity causes the intramedullary accumulation of primary spongiosa or of calcified cartilage which accompanies osteopetrosis (Albers-Schönberg disease), Jansen's form of metaphyseal dysostosis,[42] and the pile-up of poorly mineralized cartilage which characterizes all forms of rickets.[79]

4. *Modeling:* In the architectural sense this means controlling the movements of a bone's surfaces through tissue space. *It normally arises as a kind of "tune" played upon the keyboard of the endocrinologically driven growth processes,* one in which a deceleration here and an acceleration there lead to specific architectural and histological properties that become meaningful only in terms of the functions of the intact bone and skeleton. Modeling involves two subprocesses. One, termed "bone modeling," moves bony surfaces through tissue space (usually transversely) and thus affects the architecture of all bony surfaces; the other, termed here "hyaline cartilage modeling" (not to my knowledge given a specific term by any previous writer), moves cartilaginous surfaces through tissue space (usually longitudinally) and thereby affects the architecture of all bony surfaces covered by cartilage (i.e. joint surfaces, tendon and ligament attachments). This ability to control the movement of skeletal surfaces in tissue space permits the gross architecture of the skeleton to adapt to and meet mechanical and other needs; relative to the latter it also creates a mechanism which by modifying the growth process can exert control over the total amount of bony tissue in the skeleton.

Defective bone modeling produces many of the skeletal manifestations of diseases such as osteogenesis imperfecta, pycnodysostosis, Albers-Schönberg disease and hyperphosphatasia. *Defective cartilage modeling* produces many of the skeletal manifestations of affections such as Morquio's disease, Hurler's disease, rickets, and Blount's disease.

5. *Maintenance:* Here this word means keeping a bone in a state of optimum physiological and mechanical functional capacity. We probably need it because, like man-made structural materials, those in the living skeleton can wear, break, and/or deteriorate mechanically and biochemically when assaulted by constant use, by time, and by aging. One way to eliminate such problems would be to make skeletal structures very strong and massive (man's usual solution when he builds machinery). Nature

seems to have done it differently: she provided a means to *detect* and *replace* damaged material with *newly* created material of the same kind but of high quality and while the extent of the damage still remains microscopic. This permits a much less robust skeleton to last with very high reliability for 100 years or so of constant use. This physiological maintenance activity involves in the case of bony tissue the *lamellar bone remodeling* mechanism, used here in a very restricted sense to signify a special form of bone turnover; for the case of the cartilaginous parts of a bone it involves *cartilage turnover;* and for the case of a bone's attached tendons, ligaments, and fascia it involves *fibrous tissue turnover.* The latter two comprise still poorly studied and recognized mechanisms, and while in the past some have disputed their existence, clinical observation has convinced me that they exist.

Defective maintenance activity leads in the case of bone to "spontaneous" fractures; in the case of cartilage to chondromalacia and loss of articular cartilage thickness as seen in degenerative and posttraumatic joint disease; and in the case of fibrous tissue organs to spontaneous rupture or elongation, as seen most commonly in tendons.

6. *Repair* of a bone serves in the sense of healing injury and traumatic or otherwise caused defects, as well as in walling off harmful processes such as infections, neoplasms, or physical and chemical irritants. This activity represents an integrated complex which includes the basic sentences of bone repair, cartilage repair, and fibrous tissue repair. It exists primarily to allow resumption and/or preservation of biomechanical function. *Defective repair* leads to bony nonunion or failure of bone grafting procedures, in the case of tendon to the failure of tendon anastomoses, and in the case of cartilage to traumatic arthritis and premature epiphyseal closure following trauma.

Skeletal Paragraphs

At the highest level of its organization, the complete skeleton with all of its articulations, ligaments, tendons, and fascial attachments, more highly coordinated and complex purposes are served

40 *The Physiology of Cartilaginous, Fibrous, and Bony Tissue*

by integrating into a skeletal whole the particular activities we have just discussed briefly as occurring in particular bones. These higher-order functions include growth, modeling, maintenance, and repair.

Figure 2.02 illustrates the action of the growth process on a typical cross-sectional level of a "typical" bone.

Table 2.05 lists some of the factors known to affect skeletal growth and modeling.

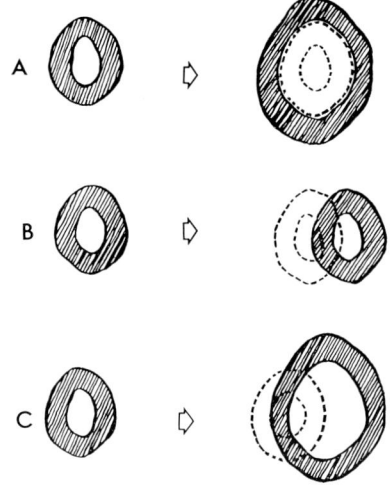

Figure 2.02. A, A "typical" bone of a growing child or animal as seen in cross section. The *growth* process acts to cause uniform enlargement and, if no other factors acted, it would lead to the geometry shown at the right. B, The *modeling* process acts to move bone surfaces around in tissue space to fulfill biomechanical demands, and does so by means of a negative feedback system in which the mechanical demands dictate the tissue architecture according to specific "rules." Here we see a coordinated motion towards the right of all of the bone's periosteal and endosteal surfaces. Anatomists call the motion of any individual surface a "drift"; the sum of all such drifts forms a composite we term "modeling" (in these volumes). Such behavior occurs typically in human ribs, femurs, tibiae, radii, and metacarpals. C, In real bones both A and B act together to varying degrees to form the additive situation shown here. This natural coincidence or superimposition concealed these activities as functionally unique and different entities until quite recent times.

The Basic Functional Plan of the Skeleton

TABLE 2.05
FACTORS AFFECTING GROWTH AND MODELING OF SKELETAL TISSUES

Factor	Kinds of Effects	Skeletal Tissues Affected
Endocrine		
STH	Increases all cell division (and all subsidiary processes)	All growing tissues
T_4	? + increases turnover	All
ACH	Decreases all cell division and all subsidiary processes	All
Estrogens	Selectively decreases cell division and all subsidiary processes	Cartilage, lamellar bone
Mechanical		
Compression force	Biphasic effect on cartilage growth	Cartilage
Tension force	Depresses tissue production	Cartilage
	Increases tissue production	Fibrous tissue
Flexural load	Leads to lateral motion of tissue	Lamellar bone

While self-explanatory overall, some of the insertions in this table require explanation. *Middle column, top:* The processes subsidiary to cell division include total protein synthesis, net protein synthesis, total turnover (likewise for lipid and carbohydrate metabolism), and tissue growth. Growth itself (and thus cell proliferation) is essential to cartilage, fibrous tissue, and bone modeling. As to the kinds of effects exerted on cell proliferation by T_4 (thyroxine), we have precious little information about what it does to the mesenchymal cell activation and proliferation processes, to cellular differentiation, or to bone, cartilage, and fibrous tissue growth and modeling. The effects of mechanical force refer to direct application of the forces named to the tissue involved.

QUESTIONS

1. Differentiate between a simple tissue, two kinds of complex tissues, and an organ for the cases of the skeleton, the lung, the heart.
2. Why can adults not develop rickets?
3. Name some first-order functions provided by chondrogenesis; fibrous bone production; lamellar bone.

4. How many ways exist in nature to create rigid skeletal tissue where none existed before? Describe them.
5. How do growth and modeling relate and differ?
6. How do creation and growth relate and differ?
7. How does the organization of the musculoskeletal system resemble a digital computer?

Chapter III

Histogenesis of Simple Skeletal Tissues

The basic structural building blocks of the intact skeleton constitute five simple tissues; the equivalent first-order functional building blocks constitute the abilities to make and to remove these simple tissues. All higher-order skeletal structure, function, disease, neoplasia, repair, and degeneration derive from these simple structures and functions.

INTRODUCTION

No orthopaedist can really understand an x-ray of a diseased skeleton, no pathologist can really understand a microscopic section of a diseased bone, and no internist can really understand a laboratory profile of an osteomalacic patient without understanding a few elementary facts about the simple tissues of the skeleton and their analogous capacities. This chapter will describe these tissues and their capacities briefly, leaving to later chapters and works descriptions of the more highly organized activities created out of them. Such later discussed activities will include *endochondral ossification* and its biochemical, anatomical, and biomechanical diseases (later in this volume); *bone remodeling* and its biochemical, anatomical, and biomechanical diseases (in Volume III of this series); *bone modeling* and its biochemical, anatomical, and biomechanical diseases (in Volume IV of this series); and *fibrous tissue physiology* and its analogous diseases (later in this volume).

TABLE 3.01

ABBREVIATIONS USED IN CHAPTER III

ENOS:	Endochondral ossification
MPS:	Mucopolysaccharide
STH:	Somatotropic or growth hormone

44   *The Physiology of Cartilaginous, Fibrous, and Bony Tissue*

Alphabets

Let us now consider alphabets further. We may well think of the letters in the English alphabet as the basic units of our own written language. Yet, computer scientists had to develop an even more elementary alphabet of printed symbols so that optical scanning devices could "read" written English and then convert those symbolic representations of our letters into several of the computer's own basic alphabet, numbers. This illustrates the fact that what one chooses to designate as the basic letters of a particular alphabet ultimately depends upon and can vary with his purpose at the moment; it does not constitute any irreducible characteristic of nature, of language, or of man himself.

The alphabet concept provides a convenient and powerful way to organize in one's mind and to explain skeletal growth, aging, physiology, and disease. In part, that occurs because of a dendritic or root-like abstract structure which alphabets and biological systems have in common. Figure 3.01 diagrams this property in a simple way, which we will have more to say about later. To repeat, an alphabet can serve to signify processes—i.e. basically behavioral things such as activity, change, sequences, and the like; *function*, in the sense of purpose; *composition*, in the senses

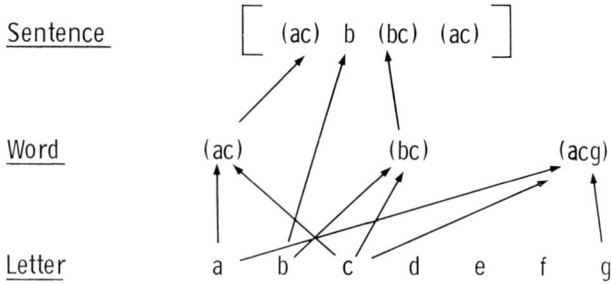

Figure 3.01. In the abstract sense man made alphabets display a dendritic structure, meaning that a particular sentence contains many words, a particular word many letters, and downward branching roots extend out of each. Also, one can obtain new meaning simply by rearranging the same letters (tea/eat) and words (Ida digs it/it digs Ida), as well as by using new letters and new words. This dendritic property will play an interesting role in devising a systematic way to analyse disease later.

of histological, chemical, and/or physical makeup; and *anatomy*—i.e. basically structural concepts embodied in terms such as "lamellar bone," "spongy bone," "a joint," "a bone," "a skeleton," "an osteocyte," and the like.

For our present needs we consider that the skeletal alphabet has a minimum of five basic letters. In the structural sense these constitute simple tissues, while in the behavioral sense they constitute the abilities to form and remove these five tissues. Table 3.02 lists these tissues, in the anatomical sense in the left hand column, and in the behavioral sense on the right.

TABLE 3.02
THE LETTERS OF THE SKELETAL ALPHABET

Simple Tissue	*Corresponding Simple Tissue Behavior*
Fibrous bone	Fibrous bone formation
	Fibrous bone resorption
Lamellar bone	Lamellar bone formation
	Bone (mineralized) resorption
Hyaline cartilage	Hyaline cartilage formation
	Cartilage (mineralized) resorption
Fibrocartilage	Fibrocartilage formation
	Cartilage (mineralized) resorption
Fibrous tissue	Fibrous tissue production
	Fibrous tissue resorption

Others: vascular supply, lymphatic supply, nerve supply, bone marrow soft tissues, elastic cartilage, dentine, and enamel

The right-hand column lists typical behavioral equivalents of the simple tissues found listed in the left column. Note that simple-tissue behavior has limited and vague meaning in terms of organ-level functions. Precisely this behavior provides the essential base for all subsidiary functions built upon them. Where naming the behavior essentially only describes it, plugging it into functions requires considerable grasp of how the system works and why nature evolved it to begin with.

Tissues

To begin, and in the classical anatomical sense, the term "tissue" signifies the following:

1. An assemblage of specialized cells.

2. Any characteristic extracellular solids and fluids with which they may have elaborated and surrounded themselves.
3. Some particular spatial orientation and association.
4. It also (herein) assumes any vascular and lymphatic bed and innervation which the tissue may necessarily and typically contain. (Standard texts handle this aspect of biological organization very well, as for example Aegerter and Kirkpatrick,[1] Maximow and Bloom,[63] Weinman and Sicher.[99])

As noted earlier, we distinguish *simple tissues* as our basic skeletal building blocks; they serve to create or build new and more highly structured and integrated entities (example: spongy bone—compact bone; both can be built of lamellar bone), termed "complex tissues," and both serve to build structures of even higher order, integration of component parts and purposes, termed "organs." This chapter deals with the simple tissues.

The term "organ" (in the anatomical regard, a sentence in the alphabet context) designates a subunit of the body, reasonably distinguishable on anatomical as well as functional grounds from other organs, and composed of a particular *association* of two or more tissues of simple and/or complex type. Figure 3.02 diagrams the organizational relationships and meaning of these terms. Such associations create characteristic and unique functional properties in the organ which relate intimately to the anatomical structure and which usually have no valid analog in the component tissues in their isolated state. For example, one neuron alone cannot think, but the brain, an association of billions of them, can (and sometimes actually does). Likewise, countercurrent flow does not exist in a random association of cells, but it does in the nonrandom association known as the nephron.

Embryologically speaking, all of the simple skeletal tissues derive from mesoderm, and each of them contains a characteristic extracellular organic matrix synthesized by its characteristic type of specialized (i.e. differentiated) cells. This chapter describes briefly their histogenesis, chemical and histological composition, histological structure, and a few elementary facts about their physiologic behavior and their roles (i.e. purposes) in the skeletal "economy," as briefly as compatible with the need to satisfy later parts of the text which discuss combinations of two or more of these tissues into new, integrated anatomical and physiological-behavioral systems or "words."

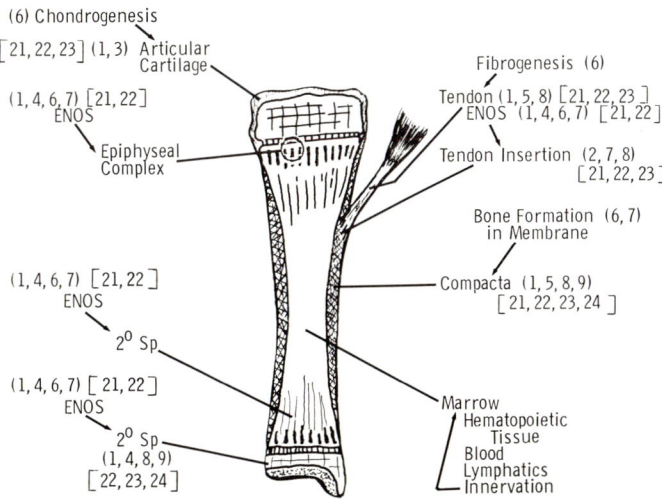

Figure 3.02. This diagram of a typical bone (here a tibia viewed from the front in the standing position) names some of its anatomical regions and lists the histogenetic processes and sequences that gave rise to them. Various chapters in this volume describe some of the cellular determinants of these processes; others receive attention in succeeding volumes. The parentheses contain numbers indicating essential *behavior* or properties supplied by the tissues in each of these regions, while the brackets identify some of the *purposes* subserved by that behavior. The numbers follow a code, as follows: *Single digit numbers:* 1=Rigidity plus strength in compression, tension, and shear; 2=rigidity plus strength in tension only; 3=high mechanical compliance; 4=medium compliance; 5=minimum compliance; 6=creation of new tissue; 7=replacement of one kind of tissue by another; 8=turnover of tissue; 9=blood-bone exchange. *Double digit numbers:* 21=growth; 22= modeling or structural adaptation in shape, size, and strength to conform to mechanical needs; 23=to create immunity to mechanical fatigue; 24=to supply a reservoir of electrolyte and buffer to the blood. The case of tendon and its attachment serves to illustrate the cases of ligament and fascial attachments to bone too. While events going on in the bone marrow exert definite and important effects on the bone surfaces in contact with them (see Frame and Nixon,[30, 31] Wu[102]), we will say nothing further about them here.

HISTOGENESIS OF THE SIMPLE SKELETAL TISSUES

The Two Major Kinds of Bone

Understanding skeletal physiology and pathology depends upon understanding some of the properties of at least two different kinds of bone found in the body (in pathological work one can make a good case for a third, termed "chondroosseoid," and briefly discussed later). While unfortunately perhaps they both carry a common name, *bone*, these two basic bone types play quite different roles in growth, in responding to physical, mechanical, chemical, and endocrinologic factors, and in pathological processes. We will speculate elsewhere on the reasons for such differences and will simply identify some of them now.

Fibrous Bone

This term signifies a biologically rather primitive type of bony material which masquerades under a variety of synonyms in our embryological, pathological, and clinical literatures, including "fiber bone," "primitive bone," "reactive bone," "woven bone," "repair bone," and "fetal bone."

Cellular, Chemical, and Structural Events: Here, as in the remaining sections of this chapter dealing with other simple tissues, we will meld structural, behavioral, and compositional factors into a basic theme to provide some type of initial *gestalt* about this simple tissue.

The production of fibrous bone begins when some type of environmental *stimulus* delivered to previously undifferentiated cells of mesodermal origin causes biochemically—but not biologically—unspecialized (i.e. *undifferentiated*) pluripotent cells residing in those tissues to begin *cellular division* or proliferation. Throughout the subsequent text and further volumes, the term "mesenchymal cells" will signify such undifferentiated pluripotent cells, while "mesenchymal cell activation" will designate the delivery of that stimulus plus the beginning of the proliferative response to it.

Parenthetically, although we currently understand little about the physiology of the mesenchymal cell activation process, we now know that it and the differentiation process coming up in a moment play vital and basic roles in the processes of growth, development, and the normal turnover of skeletal tissue in aging and in a major fraction of our diseases; in my opinion, at least, they offer one of the most promising areas for future basic cellular research in the whole field of skeletal physiology (Frost,[33, 34] Hall[44]), and such research promises far more drastic changes and escalation of medical practice and therapeutic capability than research in any other single area now defined in the medical basic sciences.

While proliferation of capillaries as well as of some supporting cells follows the activation process, we will concentrate here on the cells directly responsible for producing fibrous bone, keeping in mind that Dr. Jose Trueta of Oxford may well prove correct in suspecting that ultimately most of them derive from endothelial cells of the capillaries. Of the products of the aforesaid cell division, two groups of daughter cells arise with vastly differing fates, activities, and purposes. Some kind of sorting process segregates them. These groups are made up of the following:

1. One group of daughter cells retaining the pluripotent potentiality of its parents, thereby maintaining in the tissue the capability for future elaboration of additional specialized cells. Some cytologists signify this as the process of "maintaining the stem cell line," their use of stem cell signifying a reasonably close equivalent of the present mesenchymal cell.

2. Another group of daughter cells, which then *differentiate*, meaning that first they cease further cell division activity, at least for practical purposes, and second they begin to manifest and concentrate on a few highly specialized internal biochemical activities. These activities include the intracellular synthesis and excretion into their immediate extracellular environment of two mucopolysaccharides (MPS), *chondroitin sulphates A and B,* and the intracellular synthesis and excretion into the extracellular environment of *tropocollagen molecules,* which then polymerize outside the cell to form the crystalline fibrous protein, *collagen.* These two classes of organic substances combine in both the physical and chemical senses apparently after extrusion outside

the cell membrane to produce the extracellular *organic matrix* of fibrous bone. In the operational view, production of that matrix identifies the cells which made it as osteoblasts, and Figure 3.03 shows typical examples.

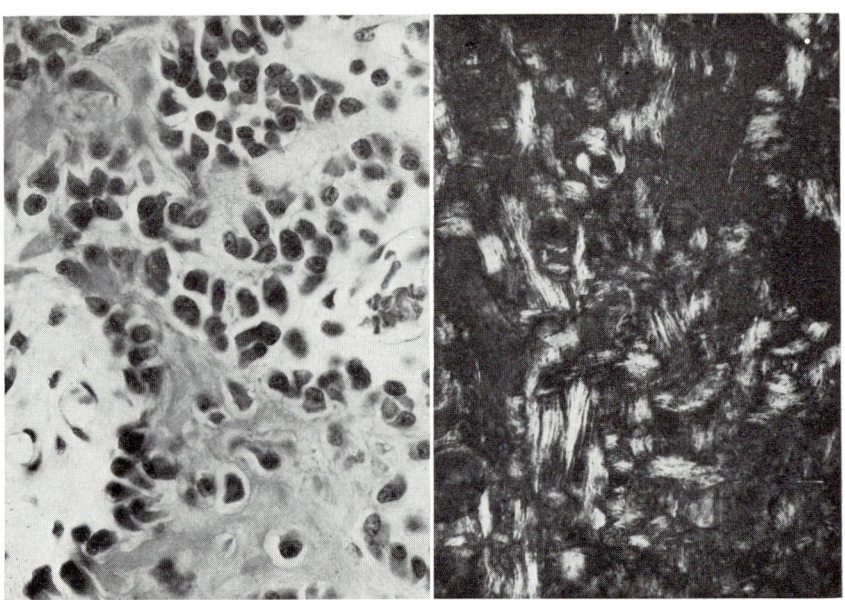

Figure 3.03. Left: Photomicrograph of stained, decalcified section of bone prepared from a biopsy at a site of pathological fracture in one of my patients (about 500x). Monolayers of osteoblasts are busy making new fibrous bone trabeculae, and a fair number of entrapped cells or osteocytes appear lying in lacunae in the new bone matrix. *Right:* Another specimen of fibrous bone from a patient with Paget's disease (case of E. R. Guise, M.D.) as seen between crossed polars at about 100x. The warp and woof pattern characteristic of this type of bone appears quite clearly.

Initially lacking in mineral deposits, and its organic fraction composed of about 95% collagen and 5% MPS, this unmineralized organic matrix also carries the name of "osteoid" (synonyms often encountered: osteoid border, osteoid seam, preosseous zone). In life, unmineralized osteoid represents approximately 40 per cent organic constituents by volume, the remaining 60 per cent consisting of water.

Some days (usually one to seven) after its elaboration, globular deposits of inorganic mineral salts begin to appear in that osteoid, distributed spottily throughout it. These deposits then increase in size and number and begin to coalesce, thereby progressively displacing the water in the matrix but apparently not any of the organic fraction, until the latter becomes "completely" (see refs 4 and 6) mineralized, so that judging by work reported by Arnold,[4, 6] and Robinson and Elliott,[77] only 3 per cent to 10 per cent of the original water remains; mineral salts displaced and replaced the missing part. As L. C. Johnson notes, and as it appears in the light microscope, the spatial distribution of this mineralization within the osteoid differs noticeably from that found in mineralizing lamellar bone.

As it mineralizes, fibrous bone becomes relatively hard and rigid and gains considerable mechanical strength in compression and shear.

While elaborating the organic matrix, the osteoblasts secrete an enzyme termed "alkaline phosphatase" in considerable quantities. An apparently similar enzyme appears wherever cells synthesize new collagen, whether in bone or soft tissues (see discussion by Shifrin[84]), so that it does not, as its discoverer, Robison, originally believed, associate primarily with the mineralization process.

Some of the osteoblasts become entrapped in the organic matrix they produce, coming to reside thereafter in small holes in the bone. The cells then become *osteocytes,* and their domiciles in the bone become *osteocyte lacunae.* A system of very small tubes approximately 0.5μ in diameter, known as *caniculae,* connects these lacunae to adjacent exposed bony surfaces and thereby gives the cells access to chemical nutrients and gaseous substances brought in by neighboring capillaries. The volume within these lacunae and canaliculae comprises together approximately 13 per cent of the total volume of the bone, exclusive of the volumes of any marrow cavity and the vascular channels (work summarized in *Bone Remodelling Dynamics,* Springfield, Thomas, 1963).

As the photomicrographs in Figure 3.03 show, a characteristic warp and woof pattern appears when one inspects fibrous bone between crossed polars. It reveals that adjacent bundles of collagen fibers tend to lie oriented in different directions and that no overall or macroscopic-level tendency to uniform order of that orientation exists.

One may write a simple verbal equation which places the behavorial events involved in fibrous bone formation in their proper order, as follows:

EQUATION 3

Mesenchymal cells + *Stimulus* → *Activation* → *Proliferation* → *Differentiation* → *Matrix synthesis* → *Mineralization*

Remember that basic sequence; it crops up again and again in skeletal physiology and pathophysiology (as I will take some pains to drive home), it explains much, and yet it has received little attention in discussions of various studies or in experimental design.

Note, too, that when fibrous bone appears during diseases such as Paget's disease, traumatic myositis ossificans, myositis ossificans progressiva, fracture healing, or in the subchondral bone of an osteoarthritic joint, this represents purely and simply the perfectly normal produce of perfectly normal fibrous osteoblasts, exactly similar in their biochemistry and behavior to such osteoblasts found in all other perfectly normal circumstances. Thus, understanding these diseases well enough to cure them forms more a problem of learning to understand *why mesenchymal cells put those osteoblasts there in the first place* than of why they make bone after their arrival. Time and time again I see my colleagues failing to grasp that simple point and going off on therapeutic tangents directed at suppressing those osteoblasts. That success would be pyrrhic, for it would suppress *all other normal osteoblasts, too,* leading to numerous skeletal fractures or it would interfere with mineralization of the new osteoid they make to cause a generalized and likely disabling osteomalacia.

Functions of Fibrous Bone

Let us list seven such functions below:

1. The ability to manufacture fibrous bone endows the body with the primal step of one of the only two processes known in all of nature for creating new bony tissue where none existed before (a high-order function).

2. It plays an essential role in the longitudinal growth of bones, as well as in pathological activities such as fracture repair, Paget's disease (See Fig. 3.03), and defense-type responses of the skeleton to harmful processes—for example, infection, physical microdamage, and metastatic malignancy (again, high-order functions). This role represents the fact that it provides the base needed for the initial deposition throughout the skeleton of lamellar bone; the latter for some peculiar reason does not deposit except on preexisting bone of some kind. (Parenthetically, my current hunch on this holds that the effects of mechanical stress on the underlying bone orders the polymerization process to produce lamellar bone, and until a rigid bony material already exists, such stress cannot give rise to the specific and causative surface phenomena that cause that ordering of polymerization.)

3. From a variety of observations of reasonably healthy tissues I infer that fibrous bone constitutes its own inherent and seemingly self-sufficient stimulus to its subsequent removal and replacement by lamellar bone (described below and a first-order function). Certainly that replacement plays an essential role in longitudinal growth, in embryonic bone formation in membrane, and in bone repair.

4. Fibrous bone deposits in the form of irregular trabeculae whose geometry and alignment relative to each other and to any underlying and preexisting structures does not follow local mechanical force trajectories. Primarily, the spatial disposition and orientation of the capillaries, whose elaboration always precedes the appearance of fibrous bone, determines the spatial orientation of fibrous bone trabeculae, and mechanical factors arising from gravity and muscle pull and acting directly on the bone-forming

54 The Physiology of Cartilaginous, Fibrous, and Bony Tissue

process seemingly have little to do with it. This forms one major difference between fibrous and lamellar bone physiology.

5. Malignant tumors of fibrous bone osteoblasts exist. Two presently recognized varieties include the true osteogenic sarcoma with a mortality approaching 100 per cent, and the parosteal osteosarcoma, with a mortality of about 50 per cent (I have learned to recognize a third, also with approximately 50 per cent survival statistics, but with distinctive histologic features and which usually arises within the bone rather than parosteally).

6. Fibrous bone production resists the regulatory effects of most endocrinological and nutritional factors that do exert pronounced regulatory actions on lamellar bone physiological activity. For example, where adrenal corticosteroids and estrogens routinely depress lamellar bone production (not their only skeletal effects, please take note and remember), they exert little effect on fibrous bone production, for example, as one observes it in fracture callus, in Paget's disease, or in osteosarcomas, a not too well appreciated but amply demonstrated clinical fact. We do not yet know if such effects represent direct action of such agents on the osteoblasts or on their mesenchymal cell precursors, although I suspect the latter to be the case.

7. It forms the major contribution to normal fracture repair. Experience with and studies of the AO plate technique (particularly study of material shown to me by Dr. Dieter Wilde of Hanover, West Germany) indicate that under special therapeutic circumstances one can achieve good fracture repair without this step. Consequently, one cannot consider it truly essential to the bone repair process, but for those of us who seldom use that plate it remains essential.

Disease

Two things apply here. First, the diseases of all of the simple tissues represent some defect in fulfilling their basic functions. Thus, the analytical inverse of their functions represents their malfunctions. Second, in the vast majority of diseases in which disturbed fibrous bone physiology occurs, that disturbance represents abnormal rates and/or locations of production and removal rather than the manufacture of a chemically abnormal kind of product. That point has sufficient importance and generality that the device of subsequent repetition will serve to reenforce it.

Lamellar Bone

Generalities

Like fibrous bone, this too represents a tissue composed of an extracellular organic matrix secreted by differentiated cells which arose from prior mesenchymal cell activation and proliferation. The details of these events and processes differ in several significant aspects from those of fibrous bone production. In particular, lamellar bone production occurs in discrete "packets" (Frost[36]), and the amount of bone made per packet varies in meaningful ways in health and disease (Arnold et al[4, 5]). We will defer these matters now and return to them later, partly in later chapters of this volume, but mostly in the next two volumes of this series. For the moment we will outline a useful but simplified operational concept of lamellar bone formation which temporarily omits a number of biologically important preliminaries. Much valuable information has been obtained about lamellar bone behavior and dynamics in the past 15 years by the use of tissue time-markers in the hands of numerous investigators (Amprino and Marotti,[2] Lee,[57] Haas et al,[43] Marotti,[60] Meunier et al,[67, 68] Jee et al,[51] and the author,[36] as well as many others). Interestingly, at least two diseases exist which seem to represent disturbed polymerization of lamellar bone tropocollagen molecules outside the osteoblasts. Baker[9] termed one of them "fibrogenesis imperfecta ossium," and it represents a kind of osteomalacia. We have seen four examples of the second in children (courtesy of H. Gillis, M.D.; J. Prendergast, M.D.; R. Wiener, M.D.; and C. Lucas, M.D.) but have not yet reported them as such. These diseases interest us first because they represent examples in which osteoblasts produce an abnormal product and second because of their rarity. In other words, *the vast majority of bone diseases represent osteoblasts producing perfectly normal products but in abnormal locations and/or at abnormal speeds and/or in abnormal amounts.*

It is assumed that the details of activation, proliferation, differentiation, and matrix formation parallel those described for fibrous bone closely enough not to need detailed repetition here.

Composition

The chemical composition of the organic matrix of lamellar bone differs in no *known* way from that of fibrous bone (Gong et al[40]), i.e. it contains collagen (95%), chondroitin sulfates A and B (5%), and small amounts of keratin. I qualify that statement because as far as I know no biochemist has yet compared quantitative analyses of fibrous and lamellar bone; none of them so far has learned enough "bone biology" to realize that two functionally different kinds of bone exist and that consequently this forms a significant problem deserving of a chemist's attention. The interdisciplinary communication barrier again, part of which arises in the complaint recorded (gently, I hope) in the next-to-last paragraph of Chapter X. Be that as it may, a whole new degree of overall order appears in the spatial orientation of the collagen fibrils of lamellar bone, such that distinct layers or *lamellae* arise. Between crossed polars the even ones remain dark (the *isotropic lamellae*) and the odd ones, bright (the *anisotropic lamellae*), as one rotates the stage (see Fig. 3.04). This order extends through the whole local region so that, even centimeters distant from a given point, the lamellae remain parallel in sum to those at that original point.

Osteocytes

As with fibrous bone, the new organic matrix surrounds some of the osteoblasts, making it so that they come to lie in osteocyte lacunae. A number of canaliculae (50 to 100) connect these lacunae to a neighboring bone surface, always that surface on which lay the original osteoblasts from which they came. As Wasserman and Talmage[93] have observed in a variety of ways and vehicles, the canalicular network affords the cells access to

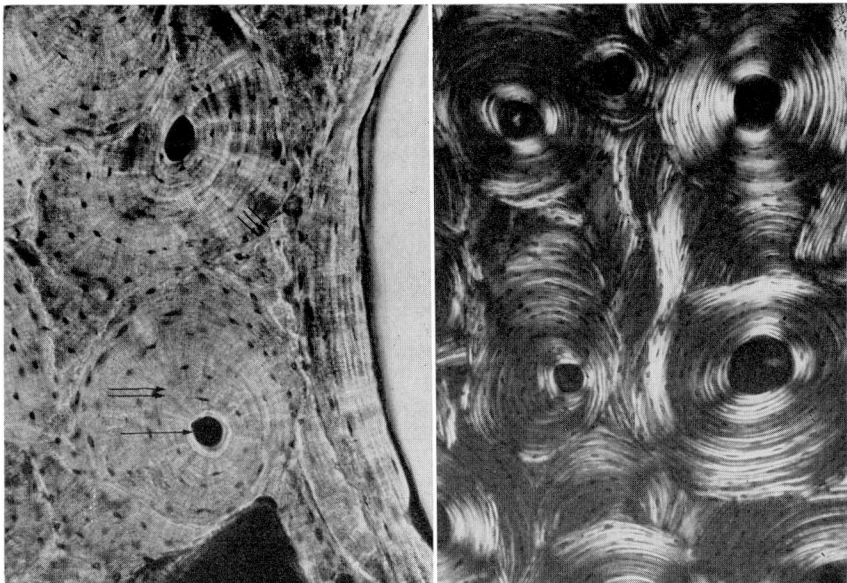

Figure 3.04. Left: A photomicrograph in ordinary bright-field microscopy of an undecalcified section of cortical bone from a rib biopsy of a patient of B. Frame, M. D. It reveals haversian canals (single arrow), haversian systems (double arrows), and cementing or reversal lines (triple arrows) (about 200x). *Right:* Another field of a similar sample but seen between crossed polars. The dark bands consist of isotropic lamellae, the bright ones of the anisotropic ones, and they retain that identity during rotation of the specimen. Both fields show examples of lamellar bone.

blood-borne nutrients. This seems a necessary provision for proper osteocyte nutrition in both the fibrous and lamellar types of bone, because the hormonal, chemical, and gaseous substances necessary for cellular survival cannot diffuse through mineralized bone itself in quantities sufficient to maintain the life of the cell (Marshall,[61] Marshall and Onkelin[62]). This occurs because, as I pointed out in 1958, normally mineralized bone acts like a *molecular sieve*, barring the diffusion of large molecules but permitting diffusion of small ones. This will become an important and meaningful fact in Volume IV, where we will discuss some probable osteocyte functions.

58 *The Physiology of Cartilaginous, Fibrous, and Bony Tissue*

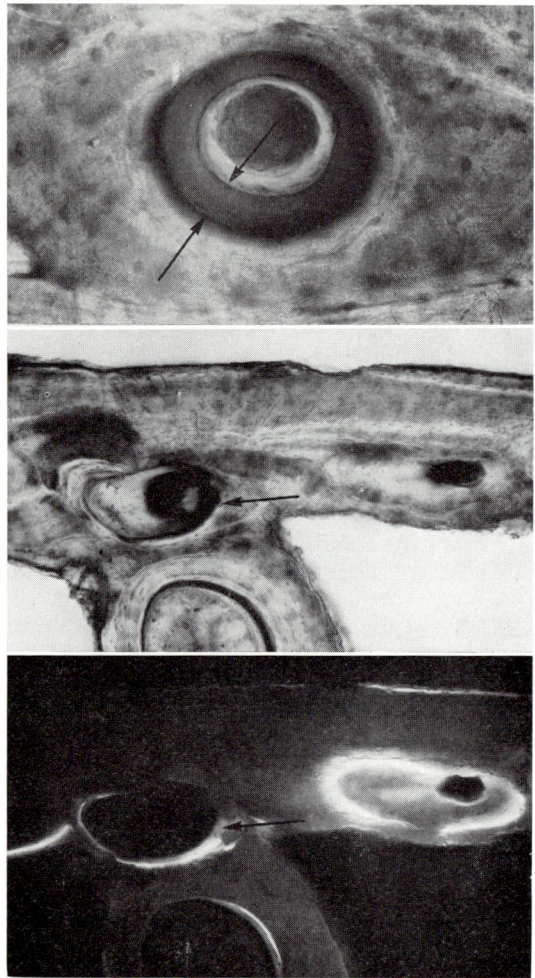

Figure 3.05. Top: A cross section of a rib biopsy of a patient of D. C. Mitchell, M. D. (About 500x , undecalcified, bright-field microscopy.) The arrows bracket an osteoid seam. Osteoblasts on its inner surface (dimly seen here) deposit new bone matrix, while the older osteoid at the margin of the lower left arrow commences to mineralize. The circular mass within the haversian canal represents the haversian capillary. *Middle:* Another biopsy sample, bright-field microscopy, undecalcified section, about 250x. The arrow points to an osteoid seam (which appears black because of the stain employed). *Bottom:* Same as middle but in blue-light fluorescence microscopy. The bright bands represent tetracycline "growth rings" or bands de-

Seams

New organic lamellar bone matrix deposits in layers, typically about one micron per day depositing on top of the previous day's layer, and associating with an alkaline phosphatase enzyme (which may or may not be the one we measure in the blood when we order that test; see Shifrin[84]). Each such increment then "matures" in some physical-chemical sense over roughly a seven-day period, following which it begins to mineralize. The lamellar pattern typical of mineralized bone under polarized light appears also in the osteoid seam, the sole exception seen by us to date representing Baker's disease, or fibrogenesis imperfecta ossium.[9] But where mineral deposition occurs spottily and diffusely in fibrous bone osteoid, it occurs in a well-defined planar region in lamellar osteoid, one paralleling the free surface of the osteoid layer (termed an "osteoid seam" and apparently first described by Rindfleisch, ca. 1850[76]). Tetracycline-labeling studies by numerous investigators have shown that it progresses through the osteoid also at about one micron thickness per day. The normal seven-day lag between its synthesis and the onset of its mineralization accounts for the normal approximately seven-micron mean thickness of the osteoid seams. Figure 3.05 shows such structures as they appear in undecalcified sections of human bone. Changes in osteoid seam thickness can occur when one of these activities changes speed relative to the other. For example, slowing down matrix deposition alone would lead to thinner seams, while slowing down its mineralization alone would lead to thicker ones. Combinations could occur and in fact seem to be the rule rather than the exception. While in theory one could also speed up one relative to the other, examples of such speedup have not yet been observed unambiguously (although Meunier,[68] and Takahashi,[91] have shown me some suggestive material), but numerous examples of slowdown have been observed.

---

posited when this patient was given a bone label of that drug prior to biopsy by H. Takahashi, M. D. (now at the Medical School at Niigata, Japan). Use of this phenomenon as a tissue marker allows accurate and perceptive measurements of human bone dynamics under a wide variety of circumstances.[36]

60   The Physiology of Cartilaginous, Fibrous, and Bony Tissue

The planar nature of the initial calcification zone in lamellar osteoid has been termed the "calcification front," the "ligne frontière" (as Lacroix[55] terms it), and the "zone of demarcation." Its planar property, plus the fact that tetracyclines deposit preferentially and permanently there,[36] provides a tissue–time-marking phenomenon which enjoys increasing use by scientists studying various aspects of calcified tissue turnover dynamics in man and in a variety of animals.

We can write a verbal equation of the cellular events and processes involved in lamellar bone production, as follows:

EQUATION 3

Mesenchymal cell + *Stimulus* → *Activation* → *Proliferation*
Differentiation → *Matrix production* → *Mineralization*

Note the similarity of this equation to Equation 3 as previously stated in this chapter. In other words, exactly the same sequences of cellular events, by the simple addition of a structural "counterpoint" or difference, can produce a different kind of simple tissue with new properties and functions.

Functions of Lamellar Bone

Table 3.03 compares some of the behavioral responses of fibrous and lamellar bone production to factors extrinsic to osteoblasts. Important lamellar bone functions include the following:

1. It provides a structural material of superior mechanical properties, one rigid as well as strong in compression, shear, and tension. Partly, this superiority arises from the fact that during its deposition, its "grain"—or the overall alignment of its collagen fibers and thus of its direction of maximum mechanical strength—parallels the resultant of the major mechanical compression and/or tension forces carried by the underlying bone. The hydroxyapatite crystals comprising most of the bone mineral create much of the rigidity in compression and shear manifested by all three mineralizing tissues: cartilage, fibrous bone, and lamellar bone. These crystals faithfully align parallel to the collagen fibrils on which most of them deposit. Thus, collagen orientation directly deter-

TABLE 3.03

RESPONSES OF FIBROUS AND LAMELLAR BONE PRODUCTION TO EXTRINSIC FACTORS IN MAN

Extrinsic Factor	Fibrous Bone Production*	Lamellar Bone Production*
Adrenal-corticosteroids	May depress slightly	Depress profoundly
Androgens	No clear effect	No clear effect
Thyroxine	Unknown	Greatly increases
Estrogen	No clear effect	Depresses greatly
STH	Unknown	Greatly increases
Fracture	Initiates (callus)	Uncertain
Given no preexisting bone	Can deposit	Cannot deposit
Malignant neoplasm of	At least two kinds occur	None known
Naked eye level architecture determined by	Factors orienting preexisting capillaries	Local orientation of mechanical force resultants
Given preexisting calcified cartilage	Can deposit on	Cannot deposit on

*Production signifies the sum of all the cellular proliferative, differentiative, biochemical, and physical processes required to produce the finished, mineralized product. The reader should not fall into the common trap of assuming (for example) that a drug which depresses bone formation must do so by depressing the individual osteoblast.

This table compares some of the responses of fibrous and lamellar bone to commonly arising extrinsic factors. In categorizing their known responses, we would like to know where (in the chain of actions listed in the equation signifying their production) these factors act. With few exceptions we remain ignorant of those details. Jee[5, 52] and Epker[27] have provided some information on this, and our group has too in a preliminary way; in this regard, however, the field remains almost uncharted, which means it provides great opportunity for young research-minded physicians, dentists, and veterinarians.

mines crystallite orientation and also the mechanical grain of lamellar bone (technically one terms that grain "stress anisotropy" or, better, even though less common, "strain anisotropy").

2. Circumstantial but voluminous evidence suggests that lamellar bone osteocytes have two important functions: first, they help to perfuse the bone with extracellular fluid, thereby making quickly available to the blood the very large buffering and elec-

trolyte reserve capacities of living bone;[37] and second, they probably somehow aid in detecting mechanical damage to the bone while still microscopic in extent, thereby initiating its repair and in effect making a normal intact skeleton immune to gross mechanical fatigue failure (Enlow,[23] Frost[35]). This operational immunity (whether correctly accounted for here or not) represents one reason for the mechanical superiority of lamellar bone over other rigid biological structural materials. We do not know if fibrous bone has the same property, mostly because it rarely persists long enough in the tissues to let us find out; its capacity to self-initiate its resorption and replacement by lamellar bone prevents that.

3. Lamellar bone production responds characteristically to hormonal agents; for example, it decreases in response to treatment with estrogen (Frost[34]) and adrenal corticosteroids (Berliner et al,[14] Jee et al,[51] Frost[34]), and it rises in response to STH and thyroxine, and probably to PTH. Table 3.03 lists some of these responses. The mechanism of that response displays special and very important properties which Volume III will outline.

4. Biomechanical factors play an extremely important part in determining the location, speed, and spatial orientation of lamellar bone formation, facts discussed previously by authors such as Bassett,[10] Becker,[12] John Currey[17-19] and myself, (ref. 33) and are expanded upon in Volume IV of this series. In this respect, lamellar bone physiology differs considerably from that of fibrous bone.

5. No malignant primary lamellar bone forming neoplasm has been found.

6. A class of diseases peculiar to lamellar bone physiology exists, examples including several forms of osteomalacia (Arnstein et al,[7] Frame et al[31]) and osteoporosis, pycnodysostosis, and hyperphosphatasia.

Disease

The vast majority of diseases in which characteristic abnormalities in lamellar bone occur represent abnormal rates and locations of deposition-removal; only rare instances occur in which the osteoblasts produce chemically abnormal products.

Hyaline Cartilage

Just as one cannot make good sense of bone physiology without understanding that at least two different types exist, so two different types of cartilage exist (hyaline and fibrocartilage—I ignore here a third, elastic cartilage) which serve significantly different roles in skeletal physiology.

Synthesis

Hyaline cartilage production begins when mesenchymal cells in tissues of mesodermal origin receive some stimulus which causes them to begin proliferating. When response to that stimulus begins we say mesenchymal cell activation has occurred. Of the daughter cells arising from the proliferation, roughly half retain the pluripotent and proliferative property, maintaining thereby the potential for future elaboration of additional supplies of new cells. Then some kind of sorting process occurs (as it does also in the histogenesis of fibrous and lamellar bone) that separates these cells from the remainder, which differentiate into *chondrocytes*, meaning cells which cease to divide and begin to concentrate on making and excreting the chemical components of the extracellular organic matrix which characterizes hyaline cartilage. This matrix contains the mucopolysaccharides, chondroitin sulphates A and C, plus collagen and some keratin. During collagen synthesis the chondrocytes produce the enzyme alkaline phosphatase. Physically speaking, unmineralized hyaline cartilage matrix consists of a hydrophilic gel, and (unlike unmineralized bone osteoid) it contains approximately (the proportions vary with age and location) 20% organic matrix and 80% water per unit volume. In synthesizing and excreting this extracellular matrix, the chondrocytes surround themselves with it and so come to lie inside holes within the cartilage called "chondrocyte lacunae." At least at the light microscope level, no canaliculae penetrate this matrix to connect the cells within it to a source of blood supply.

Accordingly, chondroblasts and chondrocytes seem to depend upon diffusion through the substance of the unmineralized cartilaginous matrix for their nutrients and viability.

Because of factors related partly to its age, partly probably to certain chemical consequences of the differentiative process which initially produced them, and partly because of local and essentially physical-chemical factors, maturing chondrocytes tend to enlarge the lacunae which they occupy, a phenomenon mistermed "chondrocyte hypertrophy" (it should be "chondrolacunar hypertrophy"). In spatially highly organized structures such as the epiphyseal plate, alignment of neighboring clones of cells in parallel register produces a definite layer or region of *hypertrophic cartilage cells.*

Mineralization

Following the above hypertrophy (particularly in growing cartilage), globular mineral deposits may begin to appear in the matrix. If so, they distribute initially in spotty fashion throughout it, gradually increase in size and number, and coalesce until the cartilage has become completely mineralized (a much better term than the often seen older term "calcified," for calcium comprises only one of the mineral substances involved in this process). In the process it acquires considerable rigidity and strength in compression and shear, and it also then becomes far less permeable to diffusion through it of some of the nutrients required to maintain healthy cells. Probably because of that, most chondrocytes in mineralized cartilage undergo slow dissolution and death, although electron microscopists have shown that the enzymatic activity they provide (and the organelles supplying it) can persist and continue for some time after the cell membrane actually breaks up. Drs. R. Shenk (Switzerland), L. Mathews (Dallas, Texas), and C. Anderson (San Francisco) have all demonstrated these phenomena clearly and reproducibly.

Parenthetically, note here that the spectrum of disease we have examined in the Orthopaedic Research Laboratory reveals that bone and cartilage mineralization involve some cellular biochemical pathways in common to both tissues (leading to diseases in which mineralization of each tissue is equally abnormal) but other pathways unique to each, so that, for example, rickets can occur without osteomalacia. We have studied three actual examples of this. While in principle the converse might also occur, we have not yet observed an actual instance.

Figure 3.06 diagrams the events and processes involved in chondrogenesis. The reader should memorize the sequences, for they are basic to all processes that effect cartilage, whether normal, age-related, diseased, neoplastic, or related to the evolution of the skeleton. Again appears this basic sequence, which we write as a verbal equation:

EQUATION 3

Mesenchymal cells + Stimulus → Activation → Proliferation
Differentiation → Matrix synthesis → Mineral deposition

Note again that a sequence of cellular events, exactly similar in that restricted viewpoint to the sequences that give rise to fibrous bone and lamellar bone, can, by varying the chemical composition and the structure of their extracellular matrices, create a totally new and different kind of tissue with special behavioral and physical properties of its own. This idea represents one of the basic simplifications and generalizations we seek to describe in these volumes.

Functions of Hyaline Cartilage

There are eight functions of hyaline cartilage, as follows:

1. Its production provides the initial step of the other of the only two ways observed in all of nature for creating new bony endoskeletal tissue where none existed before (a high-order function). That essential process carries the name "chondrogenesis" and receives further attention in the next chapter.

2. After it becomes mineralized, cartilage apparently constitutes its own inherent and self-sufficient stimulus for its removal

66   *The Physiology of Cartilaginous, Fibrous, and Bony Tissue*

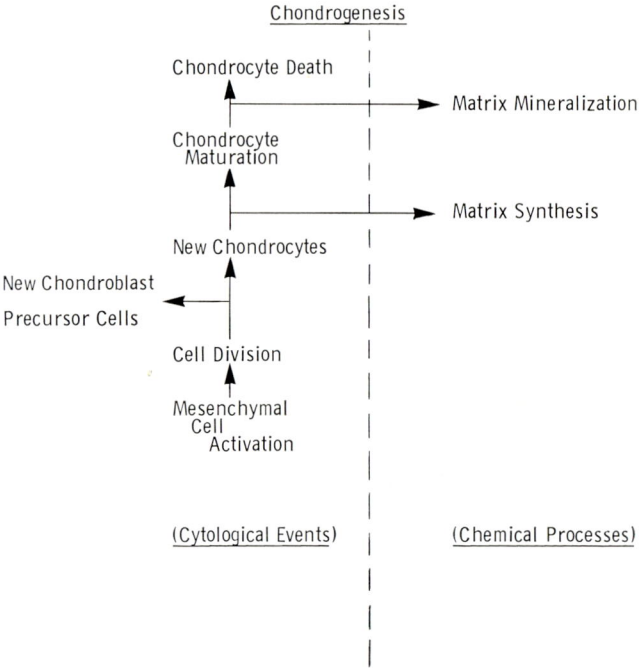

Figure 3.06. The sequence of cellular events involved in creating cartilage (and named "chondrogenesis") appears on the left of the dotted line; the initial events lie at the bottom and later ones, higher. The chemical products the cells cause to deposit in their environment appear on the right. The process of chondrogenesis represents one of the basic behavioral "letters" involved in skeletal evolution, ontogeny, and a wide variety of diseases. Just as the tissue itself constitutes a *structural* letter, its interactions with other tissues form *functional* letters, and its chemical composition exemplifies a *compositional* letter. All of the aspects in italics simply identify different faces or dimensions of the same thing.

and subsequent replacement by fibrous bone, given only a reasonably healthy (i.e. nonmoribund) individual (a first-order function). Some local microenvironmental factors can normally suppress this stimulus-property in adults, for while we readily replace calcified cartilage in fracture callous with fibrous bone, we do not similarly replace the basal layer of calcified cartilage of our joints (and a good thing, too!).

3. Chondral growth speed responds characteristically to some endocrine agents which control normal skeletal growth (a second-order function). For example, STH accelerates chondroblast proliferation, while estrogen, adrenal corticosteroids, and—to a lesser degree—androgens suppress it. That in fact explains why girls typically do not grow as tall as boys.

4. Its *direction* and *speed* of growth also respond characteristically to local biomechanical factors which receive more detailed attention in later chapters (a third-order function); these responses determine some major properties of bone and joint architecture, configuration, and alignment (see also McMaster and Weinert,[66] Smith[87]).

5. A class of diseases peculiar to hyaline cartilage physiology exists, and includes as examples various forms of rickets, the chondrodystrophies, and particular forms of both gigantism and dwarfism.

6. At least one malignant tumor of hyaline cartilage tissue exists, termed "chondrosarcoma" (H. L. Jaffe provides excellent descriptions of such lesions in his textbook on bone tumors[50]).

7. This tissue apparently makes an ideal biological bearing material because one finds all sliding joint surfaces lined with it (a high-order function). Elsewhere (i.e. Volume V), we will speculate that this occurs in part because of its high mechanical compliance and great chemical affinity for the synovial fluid lubricant.

8. It plays a frequent and useful role in bone repair.

Disease

In most diseases associated with characteristic chondral physiological abnormalities, the latter represent abnormal rates and locations of its production and only a minor fraction represent the synthesis in cartilage of matrix of abnormal kind (I do not include nutritional rickets in this group, for it represents a simple change in the relative *proportions* of mineralized and unmineralized matrix due to changes in their relative rates of progression).

Fibrocartilage

As with hyaline cartilage, fibrocartilage formation begins when activated mesenchymal cells commence cellular proliferation to produce daughter cells, some of which differentiate in the biochemical direction appropriate to the production of the extracellular matrix characteristic of fibrocartilage. This matrix consists of approximately 60% collagen and the remaining 40 per cent of chondroitin sulphates A and C, plus (as with both types of bone and hyaline cartilage) traces of keratin. The chief compositional difference between hyaline and fibrocartilage consists of the relatively larger amount of collagen in the latter. The cells responsible for secreting the extracellular matrix come to lie within chondrocyte lacunae within the fibrocartilage. Because of a kind of gradual physical flow under mechanical pressure, termed "creep" and referred to later, such lacunae after a period of time usually lose their original spatial relationships to their antecedent cells, so that the overall arrangement of chondrocyte lacunae tends to become quite disordered in this type of cartilage.

Note yet again that the same basic cellular sequences lead to the production of this material:

EQUATION 4

Mesenchymal cells + Stimulus → Activation → Proliferation Differentiation → Matrix synthesis

This equation differs from Equation 3 only in the missing final term, mineralization.

Functions of Fibrocartilage

Fibrocartilage appears to subserve the needs of pressure pads, which accept compression loads from the bone on one side of an articulation and transmit it across some type of a joint to the bone on the other side. In this process the *tensile rigidity* (and strength) but *flexural flexibility* of the fibrocartilage plays a definite role, for by adapting to their surface contours it allows opposing poorly fitting parts and/or constantly changing contours and alignment to transfer mechanical loads from one to the other, without unduly concentrating those loads on small regions of the underlying bone. Such concentrations could cause excessive joint surface wear (often seen in knees several years postmenisectomy) and even bone pain.

Fibrous Tissue

This tissue arises when mesenchymal cells of mesodermal origin receive some stimulus which makes them begin to proliferate. Of the resulting daughter cells, approximately half retain the pluripotent and proliferative potential. By means of some kind of sorting process, the remaining daughter cells cease further cell division, differentiate, and begin to produce extracellular collagen and a specific mucopolysaccharide different from those found in bone, cartilage, and tooth, termed "*hyaluronic acid.*" The tropocollagen molecules polymerize outside the fibroblasts into fibrils, and the latter assemble into fibers. This collagen also combines physically and chemically with the hyaluronic acid, also apparently outside of the cell membrane. Alkaline phosphatase appears in considerable quantities during this collagen production, both in normal and in pathological states.

We can write the equation for these events as follows:

EQUATION 4

Mesenchymal cells + *Stimulus* → *Activation* → *Proliferation* → *Differentiation* → *Matrix synthesis*

Note: Exactly the same sequence formed fibrocartilage, unmineralized bone matrix of both the fibrous and lamellar types, and unmineralized hyaline cartilage.

Functions of Fibrous Tissue

1. Fibrous tissue provides mechanical strength and rigidity when loaded in tension, but it allows flexibility in compression, shear, torque, and bending, properties which we will discuss in a later chapter and in a later volume (and its first-order function). Such properties can serve to make threads and ropes (as in tendons). When woven together properly, such threads make per-

70   *The Physiology of Cartilaginous, Fibrous, and Bony Tissue*

fectly good biological fabrics (such as investing fascia and interosseous membranes). Without such fabrics, muscles—at least of the size we depend on every moment of our lives—could not exist, for nothing would bind their various fibers together, end-to-end as well as side-to-side, to summate and transmit their individual contractile pulls.

2. Fibrous tissue exhibits characteristic responses to mechanical forces, responses involved in determining the architecture and size of fibrous tissue organs (second- and third-order functions). These responses also vary in particular ways during aging and in disease.

3. Production of fibrous tissue in the form of scar represents a major element in the repair of injury and defense from noxious processes in all soft tissues.

Disease

When abnormal fibrous tissue production characterizes a disease, it usually does so in the sense of producing too much or too little and in the wrong anatomical places; rarely does an abnormal kind of collagen represent the basic behavioral abnormality.

Note: The above five tissue types represent an essential part of the manufacturing alphabet in which nature wrote the story of the skeleton. We have not dealt here with another tissue, the omission of which some pathologists may have noted by now: chondroosseoid. Later chapters will consider some of the skeletal "words" or complex tissues constructed with this alphabet, words which play important roles in their own right in the physiology and disease of the skeleton.

Table 3.04 lists some of the characteristic roles of the skeletal tissues, according to level of organization.

THE SIGNIFICANCE OF RESORPTION

The preceding pages outlined five biological phenomena essential to the development and maintenance of the vertebrate bony skeleton. While each appears different from the others in some

TABLE 3.04
OVERALL SKELETAL ORGANIZATION

Anatomical Level of Organization	Physiological Functions Manifested	Physiological Level of Organization
Skeletal-level (i.e. skeleton)—paragraphs	Mechanical strength, stability, mobility, and power, limb alignment	Skeletal-level functions
Organ-level (single bone)— sentences	Growth Modeling Maintenance Repair Hematopoiesis	Organ-level functions
Complex tissues (words)	Creation Growth Structural movement in tissue space Turnover Replacement	Complex tissue functions
Simple tissues (letters)	Production Removal	Simple tissue functions

This table matches function and level of physiological organization to the anatomical organizational ladder of the skeleton.

respects, nevertheless, all possess this common property: each represents the *production* of a special type of tissue.

A fundamentally new potentiality was added to the physiology and pathophysiology of skeletal tissues, apparently somewhere near the Cambrian era of geologic time, by the simple addition of the *capacity to resorb* or to remove simple and complex skeletal tissues after deposition. This resorptive activity or function usually occurs in physically and temporally discrete "packets" of near microscopic size, provided as the consequence of the coordinated activities of clusters of new types of differentiated cells (see Goss[41] for ideas related to packets and biological organization, also Polanyi[71]). Now, to gain at least a vague idea of what resorption means in the evolution of biological structural materials, look for a moment at a tree. A tree represents an organism totally incapable of such resorption in its normal growth and physiological activities. As a result, its cambium layer beneath the bark must add a new layer of wood or a "growth ring" every year, very probably (in the sense of purpose) to maintain mechanically sound, fatigue-free external surface fibers of wood so it can withstand the occasionally considerable flexural loads induced by onslaughts of the elements, small children, and winds. This annual growth ring causes trees to continue to enlarge in diameter as long as they live, and so they do not exhibit the property of maturity in growth that man displays. In analogous fashion, sharks and lampreys exemplify animal species which also lack the capacity for skeletal resorption, which therefore continue to grow as long as they live, and which furthermore have *solid skeletal members rather than hollow ones.*

Contemporary vertebrate bony skeletons grow to some predetermined size and then cease growing (many species of dinosaurs may not have done so). Subsequently, they maintain an optimum state of mechanical efficiency by removing older (and presumably mechanically somewhat defective) tissue in small moieties or packets, employing the resorptive potentiality just referred to; they then replace those packets with packets of newly created, fresh, and mechanically sound tissue.

Adding a capacity to resorb to the ability to produce a skeletal tissue created two new skeletophysiological phenomena or activities, previously unknown throughout the biosphere and over vast reaches of the earth's history. One consists of a particular kind of turnover of tissue, signified in that very special sense by the word "remodeling" in these texts and dealt with as it applies to bony tissue in Volume III; the other consists of *replacement* of one kind of tissue with another, a most important activity which, although absolutely essential to the production of all living forms of bony skeletons (no lamellar bone can exist without it), has not yet received a specific name or achieved recognition as a specific, unique, and important physiological activity by anatomists, embryologists, or pathologists.

The addition of the resorptive capacity also made it possible to produce rather complicated architectural shapes early on in the embryology of growing skeletons and then to maintain these shapes, essentially unchanged proportionally speaking, while growth increased the bone in absolute size by a factor greatly exceeding 100 between the third month of intrauterine life and skeletal maturity, and while many of the various structures actually attached to it (such as ligaments and tendons) move as much as several centimeters in tissue space.

As a penalty for the benefit of allowing constant tissue renewal without its concomitant constant enlargement in mass, this new resorptive capacity created new kinds of potential weaknesses or skeletal diseases. Since resorptive activity plays a major and essential role in the architectural skeletal adaptations that occur during growth and in the skeletal turnover which continues throughout life, it should not surprise one to find skeletal diseases which arise from aberrations in these capacities, both in terms of metabolic bone disease (Heaney[47]) and neoplasia (Shifrin,[85] and Jaffe's[50]). Examples of diseases in which this resorption plays an essential role (meaning they could not arise if no skeletal resorption occurred) would include all acquired forms of osteoporosis, all fatigue failures of bone and fibrous tissues, osteopetrosis, all destructive bone metastases and primary tumors, hyperphosphatasia, osteogenesis imperfecta, Paget's disease of bone, and unicameral bone cyst.

Partly for the above reasons, the capacity to resorb skeletal tissues must represent additional *behavioral* letters in our skeletal "alphabet." Since resorption by active cellular activity occurs in both types of bone, because good circumstantial evidence implies a similar resorptive mechanism in fibrous tissue, and because resorption of cartilaginous tissue can occur after it mineralizes, the text will consider the resorptive faculties to represent behavioral subletters associated with the respective structural contexts. When we know more about the biochemical and differentiative mechanisms involved in resorption we may wish to modify that construct.

Resorption of bone and cartilage display one intriguing property remarked on by many who preceded me in exploring this country: With great regularity their organic matrices do not undergo resorption until after they have become mineralized. The only exception I have seen to this so far arose in some severe inflammatory conditions caused by infections. That exception not withstanding, the observation implies that the mineral in the organic matrix serves some essential chemical and/or energic role in its later resorption (see Hancox[45]).

We can display some of the roles of hard tissue resorption in adding to physiological potential and versatility during evolution by means of the following simple word diagram:

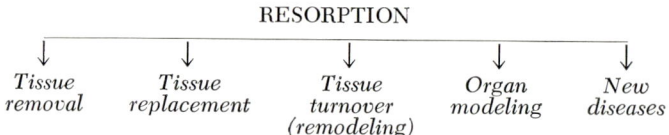

SOME BIOCHEMICAL AND GENETIC RELATIONS BETWEEN CELLS OF SKELETAL TISSUES

Cellular biology and the chemical basis of genetics provide interesting and helpful insights into some similarities as well as differences in the cells which construct and resorb the various skeletal tissues. During this immediate discussion, such cells will include those that synthesize fibrous tissue, hyaline cartilage, fibrocartilage, fibrous bone, lamellar bone, chondroosseoid, and adipose tissue.

To understand these similarities and differences, recall that we all derive from a single fertilized ovum, and that a central thesis of modern biology holds that as that cell and its daughters go through the numerous subsequent divisions that eventually create the adult body, the genetic message encoded in the DNA of the original ovum undergoes exact duplication and transmission to all subsequent descendants. A further central thesis of modern biology holds that the biochemical basis of cellular differentiation lies in the fact that most of the possible biochemical potentialities stored as coding sequences in the nuclear DNA of undifferentiated cells exist in an actively blocked or *repressed* state; removing a particular repression, known as *derepression*, can then activate or put into operation a particular intracellular biochemical pathway.

It follows that the appearance of the cellular synthesis of collagen signifies derepression of that portion of the cell's genetic message (an *operon*) which endows it with the specific biochemical machinery required to synthesize collagen. Parenthetically, Hector DeLuca on the basis of truly outstanding biochemical research has produced evidence that the active vitamin D metabolite (he prefers with sound logic to call it a hormone, synthesized via activation by ultraviolet light by the endocrine organ named the skin) works in just this manner—that is, derepressing an operon which subsequently turns up the calcium pump in the bowel epithelium (any error in relaying this concept is mine, not Dr. DeLuca's).

Presumably, the basic sequence for initiating collagen synthesis in a cell would begin with derepression of the appropriate operon of the DNA code, then *transcription* of the coding sequences in that operon into specific species of *messenger RNA*, which then leave the nucleus, fasten to *ribosomes* in the cytoplasm, and with the aid of *transfer RNA* (which brings in particular amino acids as required and as Jacob and Monod postulated[49]), then assembles the basic tropocollagen molecule, thereby *translating* the original DNA coding sequences into specific amino acid sequences in a polypeptide chain.

In the case of MPS, a slightly different sequence probably exists. Here one species of proteins assembled on the ribosomes probably form in part the protein backbone; and another species, the enzymes which will actually synthesize the mucopolysaccharides. At present the macromolecular sequences involved in mucopolysaccharide synthesis remain quite unclear, and so we will spend no further time on that aspect of their chemistry (see Fig. 3.07).

In the light of the above it becomes meaningful that all of the simple skeletal tissues named (we omit discussion of teeth and elastic cartilage here, and traces of keratin) contain only two different classes of extracellular but nevertheless organic and thus cellularly synthesized substances. The first represents the crystalline protein, collagen, which all of them have in common; the second, MPS. While the collagen appears to comprise a common chemical and structural denominator in all of these tissues, the MPS in them differ *in ways characteristic of each tissue.* Thus, in fatty, connective, and fibrous tissues one finds primarily hya-

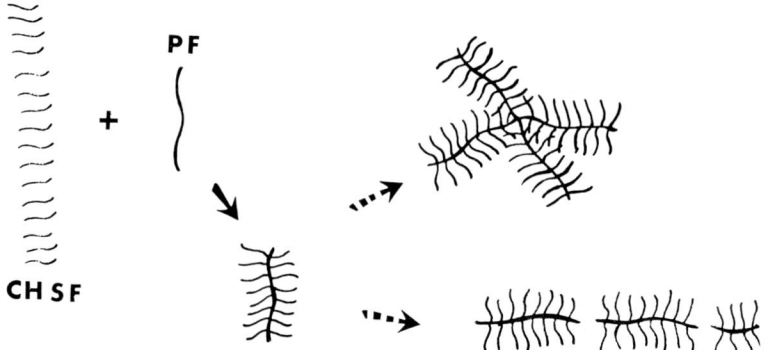

Figure 3.07. Relatively recent studies have unraveled some of the structural mysteries of MPS chemistry. The hydrophilic chondroitin sulfate chain fragments (CHSF) bond at one end to a protein fragment backbone (PF) to produce a structure resembling a test-tube bristle brush. These can aggregate by simple entanglement (top right) or by end-to-end polymerization (bottom right) to create specific physical properties of the aggregate.

luronic acid; in fibro- and hyaline cartilage one finds chondroitin sulfates A and C; in fibrous and lamellar bone one finds chondroitin sulfates A and B. This means that we can construct a simple list of the biochemical activities which distinguish the characteristic cells of the above tissues (and which also therefore determine the biochemical compositions of those tissues); this list appears in Table 3.05. From this viewpoint, *all of the cells involved in synthesizing skeletal tissues display striking similarities; their chemically specifiable differences arise from simple and precise differences in the specific MPS they synthesize.*

So, osteoblasts making fibrous and lamellar bone appear indistinguishable from each other in biochemical terms, while in the same terms both differ in a characteristic but simple way from chondroblasts making hyaline and fibrocartilage; the latter two differ from each other primarily in the relative quantities of collagen and MPS they make rather than from any differences in their kinds. Fibrous, connective, and adipose tissues differ from the above primarily in that while both probably produce extracellular hyaluronic acid and collagen, intracellular storage of tri-

Histogenesis of Simple Skeletal Tissues

TABLE 3.05
COMPONENTS OF SKELETAL TISSUES

Tissue	Characteristic Inorganic Salts	Characteristic Mucopolysaccharides*	Characteristic Protein	Innervation	Intrinsic Blood Supply
Chondroosseoid	0	Chondroitin sulfates A, B, C	Collagen	0	Yes
Fibrous bone	Hydroxyapatite, M_g, PO_4, CO_3, citrate, N_a	Chondroitin sulfates A, B	Collagen	?	Yes
Lamellar bone	Same as above	Chondroitin sulfates A, B	Collagen	Yes	Yes
Hyaline cartilage	Same as above	Chondroitin sulfates A, C	Collagen	0	0
Fibrocartilage	0	Chondroitin sulfates A, C	Collagen	0	0
Fibrous tissue	0	Hyaluronic acid	Collagen	Yes	Yes

*Some keratin accompanies all of these, but it has not yet received detailed study in a variety of developmental and pathological states.

The left column names the simple tissues of the skeleton in the morphological sense, and using the appropriate vocabulary. The next one lists the insoluble mineral salts typically deposited in their extracellular parts. The third lists the typical MPS found in each. The fourth column makes it clear that all contain collagen. Thus, the typical chemical compositional properties of these tissues appear to derive from very simple basic alterations in the kinds, and number of kinds, of MPS elaborated by their cells.

glycerides in the latter occurs to a far greater degree than one finds in any other kind of cell found in the skeletal tissues.

We may then infer that the major differences between the cells of the different skeletal tissue types represent very simple differences in their patterns of MPS-oriented codon derepressions in the cellular nuclei.

Now, take for a moment the view that malignancy involves in part some "confusion" in the specificity of biochemical differentiation of the cells of a tissue (i.e. in the precision and specificity of operon derepression). Also, acknowledge two observed facts: (a) that the greater such confusion, usually the more anaplastic the clinical behavior of the resulting neoplasm; and (b) non-malignant cells engaging actively in cell division tend strongly to suppress internal differentiative biochemical activity, while normal cells displaying differentiated activity (such as collagen synthesis) somehow tend equally strongly to suppress cell division. Then we can see some molecular-biological basis for the fact that a given tumor, for example a fibrosarcoma, may in some locations exhibit more fat storage (confusion in relative emphasis and totality of particular codon derepressions) than collagen synthesis, making it hard to decide if one should label it a liposarcoma or a fibrosarcoma. This actually analogizes a familiar dilemma to pathologists. Note that both fat storage and collagen synthesis identify differentiation on the part of the responsible cells, and that in "typing" tumors, we look typically for the characteristic microscopic and histochemical evidence of differentiative behavior that identifies their tissue of origin (we hope, but cannot yet prove). We can also see that another tumor representing primarily a bone-forming osteogenic sarcoma (in chemical terms, synthesis of collagen plus chondroitin sulfates A and B), could in some regions produce cartilage-like tissue (collagen plus chondroitin sulfates A and C), and in others resemble a fibrosarcoma alone (collagen plus hyaluronic acid), by introducing minor changes in the patterns of MPS synthesis. We can see why slightly more operon derepressive confusion could lead to a mesenchymona, a malignant neoplasm displaying histogenesis of all of these tissues.

Such a concept could also explain the nature of chondroosseoid. This tissue displays an extracellular matrix synthesized by cells of the "skeletal series" which in some regions exhibits staining properties and lacunar morphology characteristic of hyaline cartilage, and in others those characteristic of fibrous bone matrix; furthermore, a gradual transition zone occurs between these two extremes, suggesting a gradation in biochemical synthetic emphasis in the cells spanning the limits of that local region, rather than some abrupt switchover. I infer that across that region the emphasis on chondroitin sulfate C production on one side gradually gave way to B on the other, i.e. that chondroosseoid represents "confused" skeletal cells which simultaneously produce all three chondroitin sulfates (i.e. A, B, and C) but which vary the proportions of B and C from place to place so that in bone-like regions the production of B predominates, while in chondroid regions the production of C predominates.

Do not forget a fact well known to pathologists and oncologists: The activities discussed above need not necessarily associate in a direct, proportional, and reliable manner with the capacity of the cells in a neoplasm to metastasize and thereby to kill the patient. At the bottom, the capacity to metastasize appears to depend on a quite different fundamental cellular property: the ability of similar types of cells *to adhere to each other* when a mass of them accumulates by the process of cell division. Normally, a decline (probably a true and active suppression) of subsequent cell division follows the accumulation and sticking processes (Weiss,[100]), but malignant tumor cells characteristically exhibit impairment of the sticking property, thereby allowing individual cells in any mass of them to break off from the parent tumor mass and metastasize via the lymphatics or the blood. The inability to stick to each other also explains the relative ease with which malignant tumor cells come off on an imprint on a glass slide, while cells of benign tissues and neoplasms do not. We have used this simple property in the operating room at Henry Ford Hospital for a decade as a simple, quick, and effective means of expediting and orienting patient workups for bone lesions (Thompson *et al*[94]).

While statistically speaking, and in the overall view, a high degree of "biochemical" or differentiative anaplasia frequently associates with a high degree of clinical malignancy, in individual tumors this association lacks reliability, as it serves only to describe some of the characteristics of particular neoplasm generally, and to make a roulette-style "bet" on the chances of a particular patient. In other words, it becomes of limited behavioral predictive value when applied to an individual case.

SPATIAL POLARIZATION OF BIOLOGICAL ACTIVITY

In preparation for what is coming, let us expand on this previously briefly mentioned phenomenon.

In medical school most of us of necessity became preoccupied with the conventional scope of the biochemistry of events that transpire within cells and the biochemical interactions that occurred between cells and their environment. Scientists have not yet plumbed this very large field thoroughly, and it provides great exploratory opportunities for research scientists for some time to come.

However, and from the standpoint of clinical orthopaedics, the conventional biochemical "view" of disease omits entirely two extremely important aspects of all real biological activities, without which life itself becomes impossible, and which clinicians observe in action every day, and upon which they depend absolutely for the success of many of their therapies. I refer to cell generation systems and to spatially oriented or "polarized" biological activities, such as the absorption of calcium from the bowel, the production of urine, the lifelong turnover of bone, the healing of a wound or fracture, and the modifications of the growing skeleton which shape its articular and bony and fibrous tissue parts during growth and throughout adult life. I will consider cell generation systems in a subsequent volume but must say a few words about space polarization now to set the stage for later chapters in this book. Thus, were the bowel lining to transfer as much calcium from the blood into the lumen of the bowel as it normally does in the opposite direction, the man owning it would die. If no factors controlled the *structural* directions and properties (as distinguished from *chemical* properties) of skeletal growth and turnover, our skeletons would grow as shapeless but essentially spherical blobs and certainly would not resemble in any way the well-defined anatomical structures with which we have all become familiar.

This matter of guiding the biochemical activities of cells in three dimensional space to achieve useful function and structural properties, which I term "spatial polarization,"[33] has received some attention in biology, as for example in studies of why trees and related plants always grow parallel to and away from the gradient of gravity, but it receives disproportionally little attention as it applies to human physiology and particularly to skeletal physiological matters of clinical importance. The outstanding early exceptions to the latter represent the attempts of a number of past theorists (such as Koch, Enlow, Moss, Currey, and Pauwels) to account for the architecture of bones on the basis of the mechanical loads they carry during life. One of my contributions to orthopaedic basic science has been contriving operational rules which predict satisfactorily how biomechanical factors "translate" cellular potential into meaningful skeletal architectural features.

Important factors do exist which polarize in the spatial sense growing cartilaginous tissues, growing fibrous tissues, growing bones, and soft and hard tissue repair and their respective maintenance activities. They affect and involve both the simple and the complex tissues referred to previously, as well as whole organs. Subsequent parts of this series will outline a few of the things we know at this time of how these factors control the directions as well as the rates of growth of cartilage, fibrous tissue, and bone.

The reader should understand that this material only begins the task of defining what controls the growth and development of skeletal tissues in the spatial sense and how it does so. These volumes will not discuss the equally fundamental problems of, for example, why the epithelium of the small bowel exhibits spatial polarization in its chemical transport activities and why renal tubular cells do likewise. While the obvious suspect represents the geographic location of the nourishing capillaries (which provide their oxygen and nutrients) relative to the cells in question, proving that is the case is another matter for another time and another vehicle.

QUESTIONS

1. How many basic types of bone exist as simple tissues?
2. What functions does the text attribute to osteocytes?
3. What would you include in a list of the skeleton's simple tissues?
4. In terms of the initial step, in how many ways can new bony tissue arise at the single tissue level, complex tissue level, organ level?
5. Name three purposes of lamellar bone in the body's economy.
6. In terms of nuclear operon activity, what distinguishes an osteoblast from a chondroblast and a fibroblast?
7. You have just excised for biopsy purposes a relatively smooth-surfaced bony bump from the medial side of the femoral diaphysis in a 50-year-old person. Your pathologist (who makes no claim to expertise in bony pathology) fears that it might represent an osteogenic sarcoma. Inspection of the sections of the lesion between crossed polars reveals the bony parts of the lesion to consist exclusively of the lamellar type.

    Evaluate the situation. What would you tell the patient? What course of action would you then take?
8. What did the capacity to resorb add to skeletal versatility during evolution?

Chapter IV

Histogenesis of Complex Skeletal Tissues

Skeletal organogenesis and ontogeny each constitutes a dual matter: one of the method of construction, and the other of the method of delivery. The terms apply to simple tissues, to complex tissues, and to all of the combinations and sequences that produce intact bones.

INTRODUCTION

Students who want to read up on skeletal physiology typically experience difficulty in finding a text which relates the physiology cogently to patient-related problems such as bone tumors and other pathological processes, or/and diagnostic x-rays of children and adults. Peter Casagrande and I ran head on into that problem in 1952 when we began, at the suggestion and with the assistance of Dr. John Talbot of the (then) University of Buffalo Medical School, to transform a loose set of resident notes into an elementary textbook of orthopaedic surgery (which Grune and Stratton did publish in 1953). A satisfactory solution of this problem simply requires better use of the otherwise confusing orthodox terminology and restructuring in the *way* in which we present old data along a framework dictated by the relationships between skeletal physiology in the broad sense on the one hand,

TABLE 4.01

ABBREVIATIONS APPEARING IN CHAPTER IV

ACH:	Adrenal corticosteroids
ENOS:	Endochondral ossification
PTH:	Parathormone
STH:	Somatotrophic hormone—growth hormone
T_4:	Thyroxine

84   The Physiology of Cartilaginous, Fibrous, and Bony Tissue

and real human growth, maintenance, and skeletal disease on the other.

To minimize ambiguity, Figure 4.01 defines below the ana-

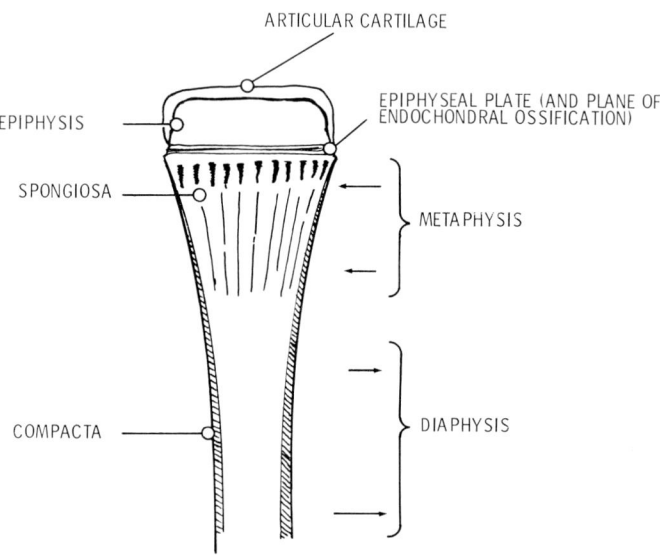

Figure 4.01. This simply diagrams our conventional vocabulary as it applies to morphological aspects of a bony organ.

tomical meanings of several terms that appear often. As the opening note, observe that the term "histogenesis" signifies those basic cellular processes which create tissues. Unfortunately, it serves in more than one sense in the various regions of medicine. In the previous chapter we applied the term to the creation of simple tissues. In this chapter we will use it in two broader and more inclusive contexts: to the histogenesis of complex tissues and to that of intact bones, which involves all subsidiary tissue histogeneses, their time sequences, and their anatomical dispositions. The histogenesis of complete bones (i.e. organogenesis) falls within the field of embryological development or *ontogeny*. The histogenesis of complex tissues lies somewhere between that of simple tissues and the problem of ontogeny. Figure 4.02 diagrams these etymological relationships in an effort to clarify them.

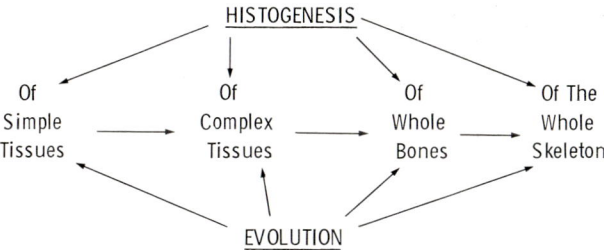

Figure 4.02. The term *"histogenesis"* serves variously in medicine to apply to problems of simple tissues, complex tissues, whole bones (organogenesis), and entire skeletons (ontogeny). The evolution or phylogeny of the skeleton and its subsystems relates intimately to those matters, too, as shown in this diagram.

With those orienting concepts in mind, then, consider for a moment the latter problem, ontogeny. Describing skeletal ontogeny can resolve into three relatively simple descriptive subproblems, as follows:

1. The means or route nature chose to deliver the final stuffs which make up intact bones. This resolves into a matter of *processes*.

2. The chemical, physical, and histological makeups of the various stuffs delivered thereby. This resolves into a matter of *composition*.

3. The anatomical *structures* assembled with these stuffs, at the light microscope level up to the naked-eye level (cortical bone and trabecular bone; ephiphyses and epiphyseal plates; joint surfaces; tendon, ligament, and fascia, i.e. the structures of complex tissues; the malleus, the femur, the parietal bone, equally; and, equally, the spine, the lower extremity, the skull).

From the standpoint of the degrees of biological organization and integration that are involved, ontogeny sums up activities that take place at four different vertical levels:

1. The simple tissue level, i.e. our basic alphabet, again.

2. The complex tissue level, in which letters serve to build words.

86 *The Physiology of Cartilaginous, Fibrous, and Bony Tissue*

3. The organ level, in which by combining the two previous levels of activity (i.e. both letters and words) in various ways, an intact, particular bone comes into being.

4. The skeletal level, which adds to all of the preceding three the additional problems of relating individual bones to each other, to the whole, and to neuromotor anatomy and behavioral patterns.

In a manner of speaking we deal here with a tree. To help to study and analyze its growth and functions we may slice it up in any number of different planes of any size whatsoever, and those at any number of different moments during its life. While the nature of the tree does not alter in changing the location, orientation, or size of the plane or the moment of sectioning, nevertheless, what we can see in it and learn about it certainly does depend on these planes and choices of moments. We may choose as many of what kinds as we wish, as long as each brings out something of value in understanding it.

Table 4.02 lists the major complex tissues (anatomical words) and selected major functions (functional words) for use throughout the remainder of this chapter.

THE ONTOGENY OF BONE

We described briefly the histogenesis of simple tissues (which provides the working basis for skeletal ontogeny) in the preceding chapter. Part of this chapter will describe the histogenesis or creation of some complex tissues, and the remainder will describe the pattern of subevents in that particular spatial and temporal arrangement that we have come to know as organogenesis, or the *ontogeny* or embryological development of entire bones. Strictly speaking, the ontogenic process should extend in time from embryonic life onwards to maturity.

In another way, and relative to the processes involved, organogenesis deals with the method and route via which a "manufacturer" delivers a finished building to the "consumer." For example, he might choose an ox cart or a jet aircraft, and he might detour via New Orleans or Paris. Two ontogenic delivery methods and routes have received recognition and names, one consisting

TABLE 4.02

THE SKELETAL ALPHABET: SOME COMPLEX TISSUES
AND THEIR FUNCTIONS

Complex Tissue	Complex Tissue Function
Epiphyseal plate (calcified cartilage)	Initial condition necessary for replacement by 1° spongiosa; longitudinal growth
Primary spongiosa	Necessary initial condition for replacement by 2° spongiosa
Secondary spongiosa	Compliant mechanical internal bony support; large surface-to-volume ratio for ready metabolic accessibility
Epiphysis	Shapes and sizes the ends of bones during growth as needed to meet mechanical needs
Compacta	Provides strong and rigid mechanical bony support plus lever arms for body motion
Joint (sliding)	To allow motion between different rigid skeletal parts
Tendon, ligament	To carry tension loads without stretching
Fascia	To wrap or encase structures

The left column lists some of the complex skeletal tissues according to standard nomenclature. Keep in mind that they originally envolved to describe pure morphology, and we now bend them slightly to somewhat more subtle ends.

The right column lists a few major purposes subserved by the corresponding complex tissues.

of *bone formation in cartilage* and more circuitous and complex than the second, called *bone formation in membrane;* yet both ultimately deliver the same identical chemical, physical, and histological building blocks and structures: bones composed of lamellar bone. However, note, for future reference, that the naked-eye—level structures made of that material generally differ according to the delivery route, for typically one produces as its final product spongy bone; the other, cortical bone. While typical, these differences are not essential, for given the correct circumstances each delivery route can supply either type of naked-eye—level structure.

These two delivery routes also play essential roles in a wide variety of normal and abnormal processes of direct clinical con-

88 *The Physiology of Cartilaginous, Fibrous, and Bony Tissue*

TABLE 4.03

SEQUENTIAL PROCESSES OF BONE FORMATION IN MEMBRANE AND BY ENDOCHONDRAL OSSIFICATION

Sequence of Cellular Events	*Bone Formation in Membrane*	*Endochondral Ossification*
1	Stimulus	Stimulus
2	Activation Capillary proliferation Mesenchymal cell proliferation Differentiation of osteoblasts	Activation Mesenchymal cell proliferation Differentiation of chondroblasts
3	Deposition (of fibrous bone) Formation of organic matrix Mineralization of matrix	Deposition (of hyaline cartilage) Formation of organic matrix Mineralization of matrix
4	Replacement (by lamellar bone) Resorption of fibrous bone Deposition of lamellar bone	Replacement (by primary spongiosa) Partial resorption of calcified cartilage Deposition of fibrous bone
5	Remodeling (for remainder of life)	Replacement (by secondary spongiosa) Resorption of primary spongiosa Deposition of lamellar bone
6	—	Remodeling (for remainder of life)

The left side lists the histological sequences involved in intramembranous bone formation from the primordial above to the last appearing below. The right side lists the sequences that apply for endochondral ossification. In this table these two terms serve in the limited sense of the histogenesis of complex tissues, and they describe only a fraction of the processes involved in organogenesis. In order to include ontogeny of a whole bone we would need to add spatial and additional temporal factors, which a table alone could not conveniently or effectively display.

cern from embryonic life on through until our eventual death. As a complex tissue represents a structural word, and a bone a sentence, the creation and maintenance of such an organ over one's lifespan represents a kind of functional paragraph in the skeletal alphabet analogy.

Table 4.03 summarizes the cellular events involved in each of those two routes. Now for more details on them, and keep in mind that at this point that we will discuss organogenesis.

Intramembranous Bone Formation

This particular process of creating and delivering a whole bone, long ago assigned its name by embryologists, involves the initial deposition of trabeculae of fibrous bone in certain locations in the embryo body and, quite important in the functional sense, without any rigid skeletal tissues having existed there previously. These locations include what eventually become the bones of the cranial vault, parts of the mandible, and the middle third of the clavicle (purists could make a very effective argument for including the diaphyseal periosteal cortex of all long bones). Typically, these structures initially arise as individual trabeculae of fibrous bone, but the whole displays higher spatial order, for instead of forming a shapeless jumble neighboring trabeculae array in such a way as to make recognizable rods (in the case of the anlage of the clavicle) or sheets of bone (in the case of the cranial vault) out of the whole trabecular mass; that mass forms the bony *anlage* of the organ-to-be. Soon after these trabeculae materialize and mineralize they then begin to undergo partial resorption, and newly formed lamellar bone then deposits on the remainder, i.e. they undergo *replacement* by lamellar bone. That itself later undergoes partial resorption and replacement by still newer lamellar bone. For the remainder of life and throughout many further (i.e. $\approx 10X$) complete turnover cycles this lamellar bone persists, indistinguishable in any chemical way or in any physiological potential from lamellar bone delivered by the other, and the next described, route.

In simple words, we may write the above organogenetic process as the following verbal sequence or equation:

EQUATION 5

Fibrous bone histogenesis + Spatial order → Replacement by lamellar bone → Lifelong turnover + Modeling

Now, if we want to write the equation for intramembranous bone formation in the complex tissue sense, we simply subtract the spatial order from the above to obtain the following:

EQUATION 6

Fibrous bone histogenesis → Replacement by lamellar bone → Lifelong turnover

The latter sequence occurs again and again in bone repair, metabolic bone disease, and bone tumorous pathology.

Table 4.04 lists some of the postnatal situations in which the same sequence occurs and explains many microscopic, radiologic, and clinical behavioral phenomena.

TABLE 4.04

EXAMPLES OF THE HISTOGENETIC SEQUENCE OF BONE FORMATION IN MEMBRANE

1. In the embryo: Gives rise to bones of the cranial vault, most of the mandible, middle part of the clavicle, and the initial diaphyseal cortex (organogenetic-level activities).
2. In postnatal life: Occurs on diaphyseal periosteal surfaces during periods of unusually rapid growth in diameter (a complex tissue-level activity).
3. Osteoblastic metastases simply represent the products of this sequence; the tumor cells in some way reactivate this histogenetic system locally within the marrow cavity (a complex tissue-level activity).
4. All bony walling-off processes stimulated by irritative lesions (infection, chondroblastoma, local trauma, "periostitis") exhibit the same sequence (complex tissue-level activities).
5. Occurs in all tumors that form fibrous bone (osteosarcoma, hamartoma), in myositis ossificans, in post-traumatic ligamentous ossification (Pellegrini-Stieda's phenomenon), and in Paget's disease.
6. Occurs in normal fracture healing (complex tissue-level activity).

This table lists a few examples of clinical interest in which bone formation in membrane occurs.

Functions of Bone Formation in Membrane

The following are functions of bone formation in membrane:

1. In the organogenic sense, it provides one of the only two known means of creating a *new bony organ* where none existed before. As for the case of creating new bony simple tissues dealt with in the preceding chapter, this holds true in all known vertebrate life forms, contemporary or extinct, which possess bony skeletons. With the greatest respect and admiration for the famous and revered paleontologist, Dr. A. S. Romer,[78] of Harvard University, I differ with him on the matter of which bony type probably appeared first during our evolution. I believe it should have been fibrous bone, partly on the basis that a more highly organized and sophisticated system should evolve after the evolution of its elementary constituents, and partly because in contemporary life forms we do not observe lamellar bone depositing anywhere except on preexisting bone, which implies the need for some initial "self-starter" bone. At least in the cenozoic era, only fibrous bone exhibits the property essential for such self-starting: the ability to deposit *de novo*.

In addition to the initial complex tissue histogenesis just described, organogensis of an intact bone by the intramembranous bone formation route involves the additional and subsequent elements of subsequent *growth*, structural *modeling* according to a controlled pattern, arrest or *maturation* of the growth process at some appropriate time, plus *maintenance* activities and competent *repair* capacity within the whole organ over all of the lifespan.

2. In the complex tissue sense, it provides the basic fracture-repair process, a process which serves also as the basis for most successful bone grafts (see an excellent study and review by Coutelier[16]).

3. Again in the complex tissue sense, much of the most rapid growth in diameter of the diaphyses of long bones in children represents serial "waves" of subperiosteal bone formation in membrane, replacement by lamellar bone remodeling following behind. From this highly restricted point of view most diaphyseal cortical bone represents bone formation in "membranes" (the periosteum

and endosteum); specifically, compacta does not represent a direct residue of the endochondral ossification process.

4. In the simple tissue sense, most skeletal osteoblastic response to noxious factors, such as infection or metastatic tumor, simply represents bone formation in membrane (i.e. Equation 3), in some way reactivated in the marrow cavity tissues or in the periosteum by those factors. That newly deposited bone, like fibrous bone anywhere else, then automatically begins replacement by lamellar bone, which can require years to reach completion.

Bone Formation in Cartilage (Endochondral Ossification)

This term also appears in two different but usually unspecified (and thus confusing) contexts. We will describe its more general organogenetic meaning first, and then its more limited complex tissue meaning. Take note, however, that in terms of understanding postnatal skeletal health and disease, the latter meaning points to the greater action.

In the ontogenetic sense: The other means or route for delivering a whole bone to the skeleton involves the initial formation *in utero* of a hyaline cartilage model or *anlage* of the bone-to-be, and so it depends ultimately upon competent chondrogenesis. This anlage, roughly and imprecisely shaped when compared to the anatomical details of the adult bone it ultimately will become but still possessing a high degree of spatial order, itself develops from a group of primitive precursor cells of mesodermal origin, first by proliferation and sorting processes and then by differentiation of some of the daughter cells into chondroblasts which secrete the extracellular hyaline cartilage organic matrix. That minute model then enlarges further, while portions of it simultaneously age in some chemical sense. Finally, its oldest and usually most deeply buried portions begin to accept deposits of mineral salts, i.e. they mineralize. Following that, two further complex and temporally as well as spatially ordered events occur that give rise to the *primary center of ossification*. Summarized here, they receive further description in the next chapter as the general process of *endochondral ossification* at the complex tissue level.

First, some of this calcified cartilage becomes invaded and resorbed by chondroclasts associated with capillaries entering the bone from without. New fibrous bone then partly *replaces* the resorbed parts of the cartilage to form a calcified cartilage-fibrous bone complex of trabeculae known as the *primary spongiosa* or chondroosseous complex. The spaces between the trabeculae, which contain the capillaries, osteoblasts, osteoclasts, and their supporting cells, arise by virtue of the fact that insufficient fibrous bone deposits to completely replace all of the previously resorbed cartilage.

Second, the trabeculae of the primary spongiosa then themselves undergo partial resorption at their diaphyseal ends and incomplete *replacement* of the tissue removed thereby by plates and bars of new lamellar bone, to become (after two or more successive "waves" or generations of this process) the *secondary spongiosa*. Throughout subsequent life, histological-level tissue-turnover activity on the surfaces of these trabeculae of lamellar bone continues to replace older with newer lamellar bone.

Simultaneously with the above, a collar of fibrous bone deposits around the external circumference of the cartilage model, and following mineralization it too undergoes replacement by lamellar bone. You will recognize there the elements of the complex tissue-level intramembranous bone forming sequences described previously.

Now, all of the above events *plus* the subsequent growth, modeling, and maintenance activities that lead to and maintain an adult bone comprise a paragraph, the organogenesis of bone by the route of bone formation in cartilage. We might write this in a word equation as follows:

EQUATION 7

(Chondrogenesis + Spatial order → Primary spongiosa → Secondary spongiosa → Remodeling) plus *(Bone formation in membrane + Spatial order → Lamellar bone replacement → Compacta → Modeling plus remodeling)*

In a much more limited sense, the *complex tissue-level process of endochondral ossification* provides the specific means for creating several anatomically different but important complex tissues, including the epiphyseal plate, the epiphysis, the apophysis, tendon and liagament attachments to bone, the adult's chief supply of trabecular bone, and an efficient supplementary mechanism for fracture healing. Figure 4.03 diagrams the sequences of events

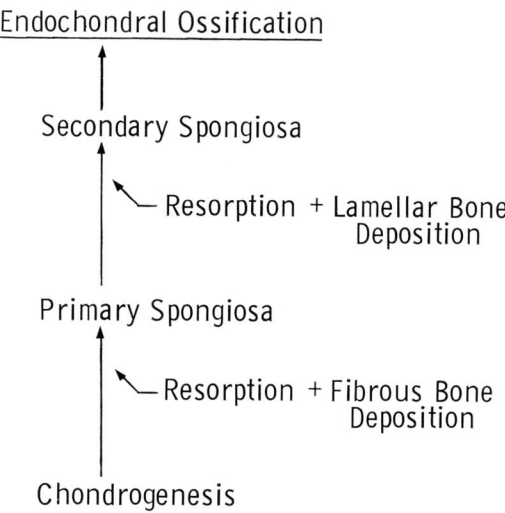

Figure 4.03. This diagrams the basic blocks of complex cellular activities that, in sum and in the complex tissue-level context, we call "endochondral ossification." It begins at the bottom with *chondrogenesis*. When that cartilage calcifies, it then undergoes *replacement* (i.e. partial resorption, followed by fibrous bone deposition) by the primary spongiosa. This in turn also undergoes *replacement* (i.e. resorption, followed by lamellar bone deposition) by the secondary spongiosa, a term that designates mature and normal spongy bone of the final and permanent lamellar type.

that in sum add up to endochondral ossification. The endochondral ossification process, written as a word equation and in this restricted complex tissue level sense, becomes the following:

EQUATION 8

Chondrogenesis → Primary spongiosa → Secondary spongiosa → Remodeling

Functions of Endochondral Ossification

The next chapter will outline some of these: a brief listing would include establishing the length of a bone, its width at the ends, certain aspects of the basic shape of the whole bone, the shape and size of its articulations, and (as one of its residues) the total amount of trabecular bone with which one enters adult life.

As already mentioned, in the chemical, physiological, and light microscopic-structural senses, the lamellar trabecular bony tissue delivered by this roundabout route differs in no way from that delivered by bone formation in membrane, even though at the naked—eye-level the trabecular structures created with it do differ obviously from the structure of compacta. So does a wall differ obviously in structure from a smokestack, even though masons constructed both of the same kinds and proportions and basic spatial arrangement of brick and mortar. That explains the appropriateness of the analogy that in the contexts of organogenesis as well as of complex tissue histogenesis, bone formation in membrane and endochondral ossification, like cart and jet, simply identify two different ways to deliver the same building (and/or building material) to the adult skeleton.

HISTOGENESIS OF COMPACTA AND SECONDARY SPONGIOSA

To repeat, the terms "compacta" and "secondary spongiosa" identify complex tissues composed solely of the simple tissue, lamellar bone; the brick wall-smokestack analogy just given applies here. In the aggregate sense they exhibit specific architectural order and easily visible and distinctive naked—eye-level properties, yet their differing names do not imply any differences in their chemical composition nor in their basic (as opposed to aggregate) physical properties. Under special circumstances a bone cortex can form almost exclusively from fibrous bone; for example, this occurs in ribs in the disease hyperphosphatasia, a good example of which E. Eisenberg, M.D., allowed us to analyze some years ago.* However, under most normal and pathological circumstances, compact bone usually consists of lamellar bone.

---

*S. Jett and H. M. Frost, *Henry Ford Hosp Med Bull* 16:325, 1968.

96   *The Physiology of Cartilaginous, Fibrous, and Bony Tissue*

Likewise, the term "spongy bone" in the general sense may signify (in addition to secondary spongiosa) primary spongiosa which arose during the enchondral ossification process, or the interlocking bars of fibrous bone which appear in fracture callus and analogous processes, such as in the bone marrow in response to some types of metastases (i.e. prostate) and in myelofibrosis. Figure 4.04 provides an illustration of human compact and spongy bone.

This chapter will not carry the discussion of such matters further; rather it outlines next the histogenesis of normal compact

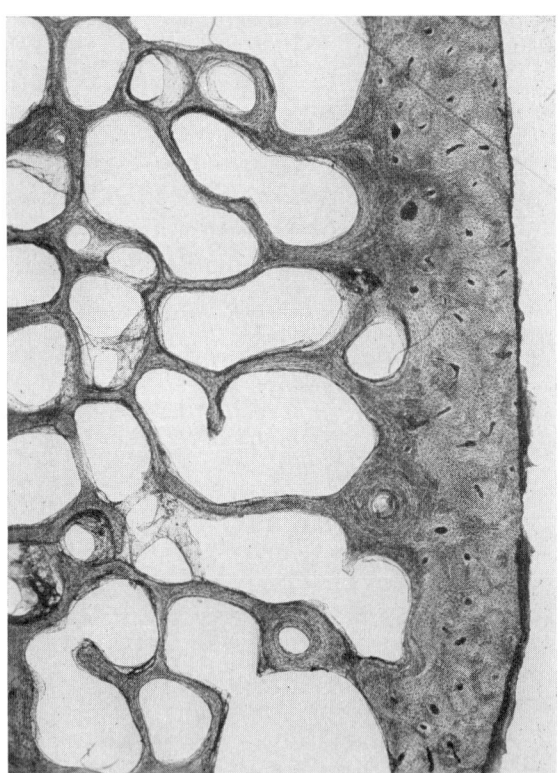

Figure 4.04. Spongy bone on the left, also known synonymously as "trabecular" and "cancellous bone." Compact bone on the right, also known synonymously as "compacta," "cortical bone," and "cortex." Undecalcified cross section of distal human femur.

Histogenesis of Complex Skeletal Tissues

bone and of the secondary spongious moieties of the human adult skeleton, both representing complex tissues composed purely of lamellar bone (a simple tissue) on which particular and unique overall architectural orders have been imposed.

Compact Bone

Compact bone can rise by three different routes, although when one examines them closely, some of the initially obvious differences in those routes vanish and one finds striking underlying similarities.

1. The first route (summarized in Table 4.05) associates with

TABLE 4.05
COMPACTA: HISTOGENESIS

Morphological events	Appearance of fibrous bone collar around embryonic cartilage anlage; replacement by lamellar bone; large centrifugal enlargement during growth, small one in adult life.
Behavioral processes and events	(Mesenchymal cell activation → proliferation → differentiation of osteoblasts → secretion of organic matrix) = fibrous bone production; → (Mesenchymal cell activation → proliferation, differentiation of osteoclasts → resorption fibrous bone → differentiation of osteoblasts → secretion of organic matrix) = lamellar bone production; → Turnover; surface drifts; blood-bone exchange.
Functions	Growth; shapes itself during growth in response to *flexure-drift laws* to meet mechanical needs; supplies strength, rigidity, and minimum compliance under mechanical compression, tension, and shearing loads; potential for repair; electrolyte and acid-base reservoir.

This table lists the morphological events involved in the normal histogenesis of diaphyseal compact bone, the chain of cellularly oriented processes and events that give rise to the compacta, and some of the functions that compact bone provides.

the external bone collar that arises during bone organogenesis by the cartilage route. That collar of compacta actually arises from osteoblasts in the periosteum (a kind of membrane), and it arises as a consequence of the following sequence:

EQUATION 9

Histogenesis of fibrous bone + Spatial order → Replacement by lamellar bone → Growth, modeling, and maintenance

98 *The Physiology of Cartilaginous, Fibrous, and Bony Tissue*

2. During periods of rapid postnatal growth, the periosteal surface may display a typical sequence, consisting of deposition on the underlying periosteal surface of a new layer of fibrous bone, followed by its subsequent remodeling and replacement by lamellar bone, and then several repetitions of that simple sequence. Note that in the complex tissue sense this is exactly Equation 5 again.

3. The third ontogenetic way of delivering compact bone to the skeleton occurs in those bones in which the original embryological anlage represented fibrous bone rather than cartilage. This includes the bones of the cranial vault, portions of the mandible, and the middle portion of the clavicle. In such bones a spatially highly ordered anlage of woven bone deposits first (where no skeletal tissue existed before), before the fourth month of intrauterine life. It subsequently undergoes resorption and replacement by lamellar bone, and thereafter for the remainder of life it remains composed of lamellar bone. Note that in the complex tissue context this is Equation 9 again.

Table 4.06 summarizes the above processes and does so also for the case of trabecular histogenesis which follows. As a preview, observe here the facts that all surfaces of the compacta turn over or remodel as long as we live, and the outside diameters

TABLE 4.06

HISTOGENESIS OF COMPACT AND SPONGY BONE

Compact Bone	*Spongy Bone*
1. Histogenesis by bone formation in membrane (cranial vault, mandible, rib).	1. Histogenesis as the final residue of the endochondral ossification sequences (in all long bones).
2. Modeling activity (osteoblastic drifts) on periosteal and cortical-endosteal surfaces (all bones).	2. Tunneling by sideways-remodeling extending into subendosteal compacta (ribs, and all other drifting bones; femurs, and all other expanding bones).
3. Waves of fibrous bone deposition followed by lamellar bone replacement.	

of bones continue to increase during adult life, as discovered and reported in 1963 by my group (Sedlin[82]), and since confirmed by many other observers (summarized by Garn[38]).

Trabecular Bone

Three basic ways exist to deliver "mature" (i.e. lamellar) trabeculae or spongy bone. (Parenthetically, significant progress has been made recently in techniques of quantitative measurement of trabecular bone dynamics; see Gendreau.[39])

1. In the first technique, and most important because it provides well over 90 per cent of the adult's trabecular bone mass, the trabeculae arise as the final complex tissue residue of the endochondral ossification process, specifically when trabeculae composed of lamellar bone have substantially replaced the chondroosseous trabeculae of the primary spongiosa. This replacement does not occur all at once; rather, in a given region it occurs gradually over a period of many months or possibly even years. As the initial complex of primary spongiosa partially covered by newer moieties of lamellar bone undergoes further cycles of remodeling, it eventually becomes entirely composed of lamellar bone. Commonly, one can still find occasional islands of calcified cartilage and fibrous bone embedded in secondary trabeculae, even in older children and young adults, as well as in bone arising in any pathological process in which reactivation of the complex tissue level endochondral ossification sequences arises. Examples of the latter include fracture repair, osteochondromas, enchondromas, and chondrosarcomas.

Table 4.07 summarizes some of these facts, and Equation 8 represents the cellular sequences involved in them.

2. The second method of histogenesis of trabecular bone occurs in the shafts of those bones which undergo large transverse motions (called *drifts*) through tissue space during growth. Ribs provide an outstanding example of this behavior, for during growth about two-thirds of the length of a typical rib grows laterally by the process of accumulating new bone on the cutaneous periosteal and endosteal pleural surfaces (termed "osteo-

TABLE 4.07

SECONDARY SPONGIOSA: HISTOGENESIS

Morphological events	Appearance of osteoclasts; removal of primary spongiosa; replacement by secondary spongiosa.
Behavioral events and processes	(Mesenchymal cell activation → proliferation and differentiation of osteoclasts → resorption of primary spongiosa → differentiation of osteoblasts → secretion of lamellar bone matrix) = deposition of secondary spongiosa. Then, turnover plus blood-bone exchange.
Functions	Supplies a medium compliance material, rigid in tension, compression, and shear; distributes mechanical loads evenly between joint surfaces and diaphysis; freedom from mechanical fatigue failure; supplies a reservoir of electrolyte and buffer to the blood; hematopoiesis occurs in its marrow tissue; potential for repair.

A brief listing of the morphological and cellularly oriented processes and events that give rise to most secondary spongiosa during normal growth, and certain of the functions provided by 2° spongiosa to the body.

blastic drifts"), and progressive bone resorption on the endosteal cutaneous and periosteal pleural surfaces (termed "osteoclastic drifts"). The endosteal resorption process (a *modeling* or sculpting activity) which accompanies these drifts frequently removes endosteal bone in such a way as to leave thin longitudinal plates on the inner wall of the compacta. On cross-sections they appear as bars and in time actually convert into bars and form typical trabeculae within the marrow cavity.

3. A very similar but distinctive third process can occur in the older mature skeleton now owing to subendosteal tunneling by turnover processes (termed "remodeling" in these volumes) arising on the marrow cavity wall of the bone, processes which remove far more bone than they replace and so enlarge the marrow cavity at the same time that they generate new longitudinal trabecular plates. Figure 4.05 diagrams these processes.

From the physiological, chemical, mechanical, and structural points of view, trabeculae arising as a residue of the endochondral ossification process and those representing the dregs of the modeling process just described exhibit no known differences. Both live in an environment that differs physically and chemically in

Histogenesis of Complex Skeletal Tissues

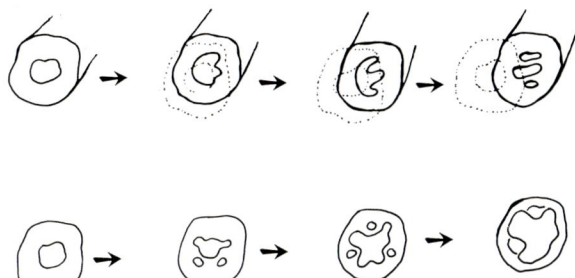

Figure 4.05. This diagrams the histogenesis of trabecular bone by means of the action of transverse cortical drifts during growth (top) and subendosteal tunneling during adult life (below).

significant particulars from that affecting compacta; as a consequence, spongy bone and compacta can respond differently in disease (see deBroyn et al,[20] Frost,[34] Arnold[5]).

QUESTIONS

1. In what regard does the subject *histogenesis of fibrous bone* differ from the subject *histogenesis of a bone as an organ?*
2. How many different and conventionally named delivery schemes exist in nature for manufacturing a whole bone?
3. How many delivery schemes exist in nature for making fibrous bone? Hyaline cartilage?
4. Which probably evolved first as life crept over ancient and now extinct seas: fibrous or lamellar bone? Hyaline cartilage or fibrous tissue? Bone or fibrous tissue? Of course, we do not know for sure, but what seems the most logical reason for your choices?
5. What causes fibrous bone to undergo resorption after its production?
6. What kinds of factors control skeletal growth?
7. You have just biopsied a lesion in the thigh of a 50-year-old person and found a thick cartilaginous cap lying on top of a relatively small bony exostosis arising from the proximal part of the medial femoral condyle. The patient originally came

to see you because she had noted the mass several years previously, occasionally bumped it, and (in response to direct questions) believed but was not certain that it had enlarged slightly.

Your pathologist returns to you a diagnosis of growing osteochondroma (i.e. benign lesion).

Evaluate. What course of action would you take?

8. You have just seen a 10-year-old child in the clinic and suspect from history, examination, and laboratory results that she may have an acute hematogenous osteomyelitis of the proximal tibia of several days' duration. Her x-rays, including comparison views of the other limb, appear absolutely normal.

What do you do now, and why?

9. A group of authors, observing certain changes in the epiphyseal plates of mice receiving whole-body radiation for periods extending up to four months, attributed those changes to a direct effect of the radiation on cellular proliferative phenomena involved in the plate.

Evaluate.

Chapter V

The Endochondral Ossification Process

The endochondral ossification process participates essentially (that is, without it, the following could not occur) in bone organogenesis; in longitudinal bone growth; in producing spongy bone; in aligning bones at various joints; in the construction, geometry, and function of joints; in establishing overall body height; in determining when skeletal growth will cease; in skeletal repair and defense processes; in selected benign and malignant neoplasms; and in the development of some congenital disorders and of some acquired disorders in its anatomical patterns and speed.

INTRODUCTION

This chapter will describe rather briefly the cellular sequences involved in endochondral ossification, that term serving here in the complex tissue sense and not in the more inclusive organogenetic sense. The histogenesis and physiology of this complex tissue form one of the elementary fields of knowledge which anyone who works with skeletal physiology and disease *must* know to acquire competence. After describing the sequences, the text will then relate each step in them to one or more known diseases and to one or more factors known to regulate it. A later chapter will discuss selected biomechanical and physiological properties.

TABLE 5.01

ABBREVIATIONS USED IN CHAPTER V

ACH:	Adrenal-cortical steroids
ACTH:	Adrenocorticotrophic hormone
ENOS:	Endochondral ossification
PTH:	Parathormone
STH:	Somatotropic or growth hormone
T_4:	Thyroxine

Before discussing the details of the endochondral ossification process ("ENOS," henceforth, to save space), we should first put it in context in the overall skeletal scheme and then specify the apparent basic functions it provides to the remainder of the body.

Context

Figure 5.01 diagrams the broad relationships involved in skeletal physiology. If we start with the organ level, its properties *interact* with higher and lower levels from embryological life on until death owing to extrauterine senescence. These interactions affect each of the three "faces" of skeletal physiology defined earlier: proliferative-differentiative, biochemical, and spatial polarization. Each system imposes its own properties on the whole complex in terms of capability and limitation. While the main direction of flow of such informational interaction goes downwards (which the heavy arrows signify), feedback also occurs in terms of the light, upwards-going arrows.

This chapter deals with matters occupying the box beneath the legend "Longitudinal Processes."

Functions

The functions of ENOS appear few and relatively simple, yet highly important. Note at the outset that its first step, generating hyaline cartilage *de novo* (i.e. chondrogenesis), provides the particular intraembryonic mechanism which, by some means that predetermines the shapes of the skeletal analages, thereby predetermines major gross architectural features of most adult bones (Enlow,[25] Weinmann and Sicher[99]). Important functions of the ENOS process certainly include the following:

1. It provides a mechanism for increasing bone length during growth, one regulated as to speed and duration by the endocrinological and nutritional factors that control somatic growth in general.

2. It provides a mechanism for moving, in precisely controlled relationships to overall longitudinal growth, the attachments of tendons, ligaments, and sheets of fascia to bony surfaces. This

The Endochondral Ossification Process 105

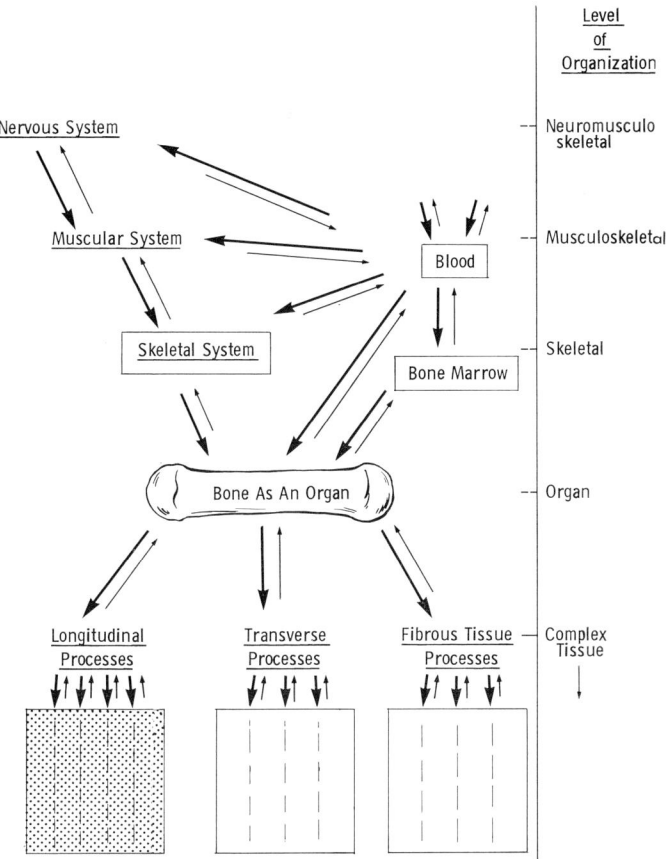

Figure 5.01. This diagrams the broad outlines of the relationships of the skeleton to the body. It represents a kind of small-scale map of this "country," which we will use repeatedly to place subjects under particular and more detailed discussion in proper perspective. Where the three faces of disease mentioned earlier comprise one plane of section in this "tree," this diagram comprises a different one but of the same identical tree.

property relates to the anatomical fact that all such structures attach to bone across a layer of cartilage which, during its own growth, responds in the same way to the same endocrinological and biomechanical regulatory factors as does longitudinal bone growth. Little emphasized elsewhere (but see Enlow[24]), this property in fact explains the development of chondrosarcomas

106 *The Physiology of Cartilaginous, Fibrous, and Bony Tissue*

at sites of tendon and ligament attachment even in adults, as well as biomechanical behavioral characteristics of prime importance in establishing bone architecture and limb alignment during growth.

Its modes of response to mechanical compression and tension forces during fetal and early postnatal life determine the shapes, partly the sizes, and partly the planes of motions and alignments of diarthrodial (i.e. moving, cartilage-covered) joints. Chapters VI and VII will explore this matter and present some new (and original) material of considerable and direct clinical interest.

4. As its final residue it creates most of the spongy bone in the adult skeleton. A simple but important fact clearly recognized some time ago, for example, by Enlow[24] and Johnson,[53] it still has found little recognition or usage by clinicians involved with skeletal physiology.

5. Disorders of the cellular sequences which add up to and comprise ENOS generate an assortment of congenital and acquired diseases of that mechanism. Some of these diseases arise from a change in only one step in the ENOS sequences, while others combine two or more changes to produce more complex and varied but individually rather rare distortions.

Generalities

With an eye on the spectrum of diseases known to affect the ENOS process, let us divide it into five substages and describe them as they appear in a typical epiphyseal plate, the drawing in Figure 5.02 representing the proximal tibial epiphyseal region of a standing child as seen from the front. (To fit the following description to any distal tibial epiphyseal plate, simply turn the figure upside down.)

> *Nota bene:* The spatial polarization or orientation of the growth of epiphyseal plates exists *relative to the midshaft* of the bone; growth proceeds *away* from that region. While it would take too much space to explain why in detail, the location of the original center of ossification in embryonic life predetermined that fact.

The separate stages involved in the ENOS process have a useful property: While the first one, the proliferative stage, seems

The Endochondral Ossification Process

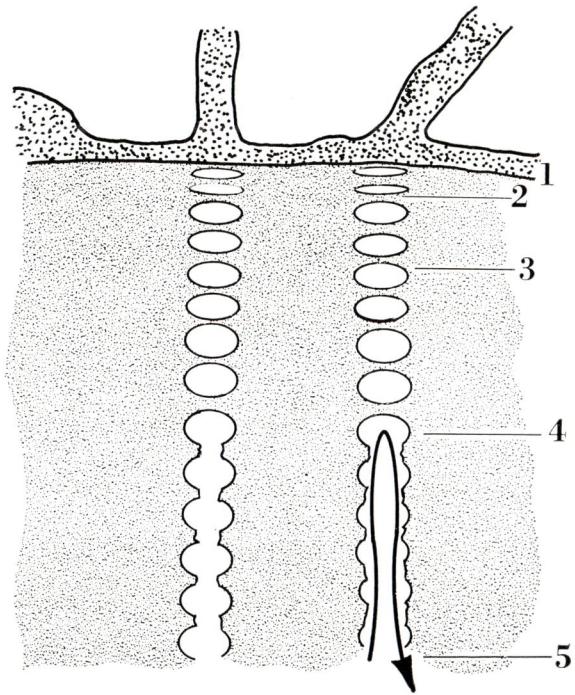

Figure 5.02. A diagrammatic representation of the endochondral ossification sequences. To place it in perspective, consider it as the proximal end of the growing tibia as seen from the front of a standing child. The speckled areas at the top represent trabeculae within the epiphyseal plate. During growth, new cartilage is added at the top (region *1*), while older cartilage is removed from below (region *5*). The sequences which in sum produce that overall effect consist of (1) chondroblast proliferation, (2) sorting of the stem cell from the differentiated cell line, (3) chondral matrix synthesis, (4) mineralization of the cartilage, and (5) resorption of mineralized cartilage. A different numbering sequence appears in Table 5.02.

to depend largely upon systemic factors for its activation and in part upon them for control of its speed, all subsequent stages appear initiated or activated by some physicochemical property *inherent in the tissue and/or cell produced by the previous one.* Paraphrased, each subsequent stage becomes initiated by (as well as *following*) the completion of the preceding one. If true, then arresting or delaying any stage (due to disease of some kind)

108 The Physiology of Cartilaginous, Fibrous, and Bony Tissue

TABLE 5.02
ENDOCHONDRAL OSSIFICATION SEQUENCE

Stages in the Endochondral Ossification Process	Factor Activating the Stage	Factors Accelerating the Stage	Factors of Clinical Importance Decelerating the Stage
1. Proliferative stage	STH, T_4, (?)ACTH	STH, T_4	Estrogens, ACH, mechanical compression, excessive androgens, removal of STH and/or T_4
2. Sorting process	Seems inherent in daughter cells of previous stage	None known other than anything accelerating Stage 1	None known other than anything depressing Stage 1
3. Differentiative sequence a. Cartilage matrix synthesis and lacunar hypertrophy	Seems inherent in the cells and a function of their age	Anything accelerating Stage 1	? Vitamin D and C deficiencies, plus anything retarding Stage 1
b. Mineralization of the matrix	Seems inherent in the cells and a function of their age	Vitamin D, plus anything accelerating Stage 1	Vitamin D deficiency, PTH, plus anything retarding Stage 1. (?) Hypophosphatemia
4. Production of primary spongiosa	Properties inherent in mineralized cartilage	None known other than anything accelerating Stage 1	Scurvy, plus anything retarding Stage 1, plus Vitamin D deficiency
5. Replacement by secondary spongiosa	Properties inherent in primary spongiosa	None known other than anything accelerating Stage 1	Scurvy, plus anything retarding Stage 1

The left column lists the five major steps in the endochondral ossification sequences. The next lists major factors affecting the initiation of each, the third those that accelerate, and the last those that retard their progression with time.

should arrest or delay all subsequent stages to a similar degree, and clinical observation verifies that. These relationships endow the whole ENOS system with the property of a railroad train, in that all of the cars (stages) normally follow exactly in step behind the engine (chondroblast division). Thus, when the engine slows down, so do all succeeding cars; if it speeds up, they all do likewise; and if a pair of its cars becomes uncoupled, the ones forward of that point continue on their merry way while the ones to the rear fall farther and farther behind. Therefore, one can control the speed of the entire complex *by controlling the speed of its first stage,* and to a limited degree we can do that therapeutically by currently available endocrine and biomechanical means.

Table 5.02 lists these five stages along with a few of the important factors which appear to regulate them. A few things merit the emphasis of separate mention here. For example, the simple property that estrogens suppress chondroblast division more effectively than androgens do (Frost[34]) makes women shorter than men (my generation was taught—incorrectly—that androgens stimulated longitudinal growth). It follows that those castrated at or before puberty might grow taller than those who are not, and in clinical practice that usually occurs.

THE ENOS SEQUENCES

The Proliferative Stage

The fundamental activity in ENOS (as well as in chondrogenesis, the immediate topic) constitutes proliferation (i.e. cell division) of the chondroblast stem or progenitor cells in the germinal region or layer. This proliferation first begins when a recognizeable cartilage anlage appears in the embryo; it continues until the death of the senile adult, although very great changes occur in the frequency of such division, as well as in its anatomical locations, over the intervening span of life. This proliferation originally occurs relatively diffusely throughout the cartilaginous anlage, but in fetal and later life it becomes increasingly localized to certain planar regions in the cartilage, conveniently designated henceforth as "germinal layers."

Regulation of Chondroblast Division

Growth hormone (STH) exerts a major effect on chondroblast division in the germinal layer, for without it that division ceases for all practical purposes. Thus, all skeletal growth processes which ultimately depend upon the ENOS process (this excludes the growth of the skull at its sutural lines, and the diametric expansion of diaphyses during growth) ultimately, although indirectly, depend upon the ability of STH to *stimulate mitotic division* of chondroblasts. This fact has received insufficient clinical recognition and usage, yet it displays a reproducibility such that it still serves in the pharmaceutical industry as the basis for excellent bioassays of the potency of STH preparations (see Collins et al[15]).

Disease Examples

Examples of disease arising from abnormal chondroblast division include those due to *decreased frequency* of division, others due to *increased frequency*, and yet others due to *abnormal location* of germinal layer activity, themes nature builds upon what I once termed "cell generation system," to which Hall recently referred to briefly.[44]

Decreased Frequency: Most forms of dwarfism represent examples, for the term "dwarf" simply signifies short skeletons, and since chondroblast division forms the primal cellular step that adds to skeletal height, any depression of it must inevitably retard growth. Examples of this type of dwarf include achondroplasia, pituitary dwarfism, cretinism, and malnutrition.

Increased Frequency: Examples include all forms of increased skeletal height: gigantism, Marfan's syndrome, and the eunuchoid state, although the latter probably also involves longer-than-normal chondroblast proliferation (or put another way, delayed maturation) as much as increased frequency.

Location: Diseases resulting from abnormal anatomical location of the mesenchymal cell activation process that gives rise to chondrogenesis include osteochondromas, either as single lesions or in the hereditary multiple form termed Ehrenfried's disease; the spurs seen at the margins of joints exhibiting degenerative joint disease; enchondromas (cartilage masses inside of bones), either singly or in the multiple form termed Ollier's disease; chondrosarcomas arising anywhere, and rare ecchondromas or benign cartilage masses arising in extraosseous soft tissues. It can occur even in the bundle of His in the heart of Dalmatian dogs and some cattle, leading to fatal heart block.

The Sorting Stage

Each chondroblast division produces two new daughter cells. A sorting process then ensues, still unclear in its details but obvious in its net effect: It separates the daughter cells of the division process into two groups with vastly different futures.

Half remain in their original location in (and thereby giving rise to) the germinal layer and retain the potential of undergoing cell division again in the future. Thereby, they perpetuate the ability to continue future chondroblast production (i.e. they "maintain the stem cell line"), and so they also maintain the potential for cartilage growth and structure (cartilage modeling) to respond to the biomechanical factors that depend upon chondroblast production for their effect. Woe unto the unwary surgeon who compromises the viability of the germinal cells in a growing cartilaginous structure!

The other half of the daughter cells remain behind, lose their potentiality for further division, differentiate, and begin to produce the extracellular organic compounds that form hyaline cartilage matrix. While doing this, any given chondrocyte becomes covered over by other more recently produced chondrocytes which stack, one on top of the other, above yet earlier ones as shown in Figure 5.02. This produces vertical columns of cells such that for each actively proliferating chondroblast in the germinal layer, one underlying column of progressively maturing and aging chondrocytes arises.

Diseases

I am not familiar with any disease of this stage and cannot state whether that reflects my particular ignorance, our mutual ignorance, or the fact that none such can exist and still remain compatible with life. Morphologically, one could recognize such a disease easily because the normal sorting process puts all proliferative activity (and thus mitotic figures) in the germinal layer and relegates differentiative types of behavior to different and "lower" regions. A defective sorting process would allow mitotic activity to appear all along the cell columns, mixed in with cells engaged in the activities of the third stage.

The Chondrocyte Differentiative Sequence

The Matrix Synthesis Stage

In the operational sense, the differentiated chondroblasts exhibit two obviously recognizeable and quite different biochemical phases to their lifespans.

The first or matrix synthesis stage begins shortly after completion of the sorting process and consists of elaborating the hydrophilic, intercellular, cartilage matrix gel which surrounds these cells, that is, collagen plus chondroitin sulfates A and C.

> *Nota bene:* The process identified in a previous chapter as chondrogenesis includes all of the preceding events: proliferation, sorting, and matrix synthesis.

Mineralization Phase

During this second stage, which under varying circumstances commences from days to many months after the first, the chondroblasts initiate in some way and then promote the subsequent progression of mineralization of the previously elaborated cartilage matrix. Since this occurs at about the same stage of their lifespan in all of the chondrocytes in the plate, and since those cells form a rough kind of planar region of cells lying in parallel register deep in the cartilage plate, the mineralization process gives rise to the essentially planar *zone of calcified cartilage,* which becomes hard and strong as a consequence of its mineral deposits and also relatively impermeable to large-moleculed cellular nutrients. The latter development probably causes the germinal layers of all chondral planar growth regions to derive most of their nutrients from the epiphyseal rather than the metaphyseal blood supply and to die if the former is eliminated but not if the latter is. Thus, in growing children a surgeon may destroy the metaphyseal blood supply with impunity as far as affecting subsequent longitudinal bone growth at the neighboring epiphyseal plate is concerned, but he must take great care during surgical bony procedures in children to preserve unimpaired the blood supply to epiphyses. Compromising that blood supply can arrest subsequent longitudinal growth at that plate. Recent experimental work on rats, seeming to contradict that statement, really does not, for matters of real clinical experience and of absolute (rather than relative) lengths of diffusion pathways through tissues are involved.

The "maturing" or "aging" cartilage cells provide an unambiguous example of a cellular phenomenon I once termed the "metabolic sequence" (it remains a good term in my opinion). As Hall[44] implied, this basic idea and others that accompanied it look better and better with passing time.

Diseases

Delayed mineralization of the cartilaginous matrix causes an increase in the thickness of the uncalcified layer of cartilage above it. When this uncalcified matrix has relatively normal physical properties, the resulting defect forms the rare disease of congenital origin known as the metaphyseal dysostosis of Jansen (see descriptions by Gram et al,[42] and Rubin[79]). When the uncalcified cartilage also has abnormal physical properties (i.e. when it becomes softer and more susceptible to mechanical creep than normal), we know the resulting defect as rickets. When that defect represents the consequence of a nutritional deficiency of vitamin D, the disease becomes *nutritional rickets,* but when it arises as the consequence of some coding error of genetic origin in that fraction of the cellular DNA which encodes the biochemical pathways that make it possible for these cells to perform their usual chemical functions, the resulting disease becomes *congenital rickets* (example: familial hypophosphatemic rickets as discussed by Arnstein and Frame[7]). If primary disease elsewhere in the body ultimately causes this defect, it then becomes *secondary rickets* (example: renal rickets).

Development of the Primary Spongiosa

On the diaphyseal or bony-shaft side of above events, cellular proliferative activity arises in capillaries adjacent to the calcified cartilage, most likely triggered off by some inherent physical chemical property of mineralized cartilage. As J. Trueta, C. Anderson, R. Schenk, and Les Matthews have shown in various ways and systems, cells capable of resorbing the calcified cartilage, usually of the uninucleate kind, then differentiate and resorb the calcified cartilage in a direction paralleling the long axis of the chondrocyte columns and extending towards the germinal layer.

We may write this as follows:

EQUATION 10: CHONDRAL RESORPTION
Calcified cartilage + Mesenchymal cell activation → Differentiation → New chondroclasts

Following a step behind this resorptive activity, new osteoblasts then differentiate and deposit the organic matrix of fibrous bone on the exposed surfaces of the previously partially resorbed calcified cartilage, now present in the form of bars with scalloped borders. Shortly afterwards, this new bone matrix also begins to mineralize. The resulting mineralized chondrosseous complex or trabeculated mass composed partly of scalloped bars of mineralized cartilage and partly of fibrous bone deposited on those bars has been named the "primary spongiosa." Figure 5.03 diagrams the above process. This portion of the sequence we can write as follows:

EQUATION 11: PRIMARY SPONGIOSA
Partly resorbed calcified cartilage + Mesenchymal cell activation → Differentiation → Fibrous bone formation

Observe one major function of the above processes: In sum they form the first stage of a two-stage process which replaces

The Endochondral Ossification Process

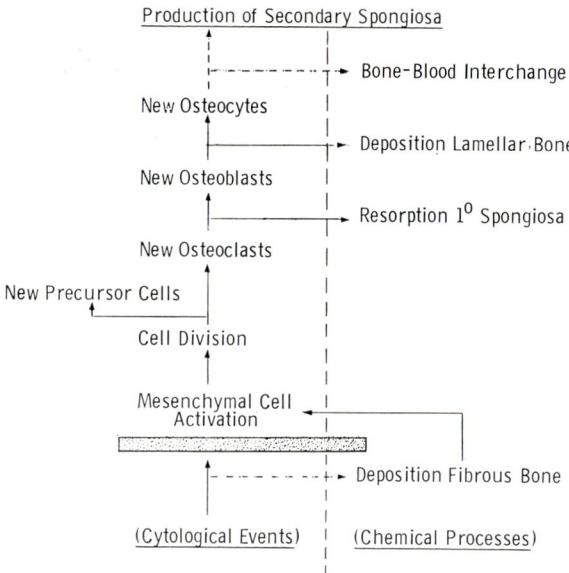

Figure 5.03. This figure lists the basic sequences involved in producing the primary spongiosa, beginning at the bottom and proceeding upwards. I inverted these figures to give the reader practice at seeing these sequences at either end of a long bone and correctly oriented in the spatial and directional senses, not with respect to these printed pages but with respect to the diaphyses of the bones themselves. Thus, this diagram applies to the lower end of the bone shown in Figure 3.02. The activities below the shaded horizontal bar (which signifies a calcified cartilage layer) represent the process of chondrogenesis already discussed. The sequences above it sketch in ascending order and sequence the details of the process which *replaces* calcified cartilage *(not transforms it)* by primary spongiosa.

hyaline cartilage by lamellar bone. Note also two other observations: Direct replacement of cartilage by lamellar bone apparently cannot occur in nature, for we have never seen it under any circumstance; and a similar replacement process may not affect fibrocartilage.

Diseases

If something retards only the production of primary spongiosa, the marrow cavity in the metaphysis will tend to fill up with unresorbed calcified cartilage, for if other things remain equal, cartilage growth itself would continue unimpaired (the railroad train effect, in which uncoupling occurs between the fourth and fifth cars). This presents the major radiographically evident defect in osteopetrosis or Albers-Schönberg disease.

When fibrous bone cannot deposit (or mineralize) as fast as the cartilage undergoes resorption, a plane of mechanical weakness arises below the plate, which makes the patient more than ordinarily susceptible to slipped epiphyses following minimal trauma. Exactly such phenomena occur in scurvy (where the inability to hydroxylate proline retards the capacity to produce new collagen for woven bone below the local needs), and in congenital lues (in which a granuloma-like tissue replaces much of what should form the primary spongiosa).

Note that many investigators, perhaps not as much "with" bone biology as they might be, make the elementary strategic mistake of studying how agents (under investigation as possible cures for diseases peculiar to the adult) affect the turnover of primary spongiosa in experimental animals. Examples of such diseases include postmenopausal osteoporosis, osteomalacia of divers kinds, fracture nonunion and healing rate, hyperparathyroidism, and Cushing's osteoporosis. By now the reader can appreciate that only by the most remote chance would such a strategy provide therapeutically relevant data in terms of the basic goal.

Secondary Spongiosa

Trailing behind the above process by a few dozen microns, yet further cellular proliferative and differentiative activities appear which produce yet other new cell populations. Some, multinucleated in type and termed "osteoclasts," partially resorb (i.e. solubilize both the organic and inorganic fractions of) the trabecular bars of the primary spongiosa; following behind them, new osteoblasts materialize which deposit on the unresorbed remainder of the trabeculae new organic bone matrix of the lamellar type. This process ultimately forms the trabeculae which compose the secondary spongiosa, and Figure 5.04 diagrams its sequences. The following verbal equation expresses it:

EQUATION 12: SECONDARY SPONGIOSA
Primary spongiosa → Mesenchymal cell activation → Proliferation → Differentiation of osteoclasts → Resorption → Differentiation of osteoblasts → Lamellar bone production

This forms the second stage of the two-stage process that replaces cartilage by lamellar bone. To repeat, this process creates most of the cancellous or spongy bone found in the adult skeleton, a fact which will become more meaningful in Volume III. Judg-

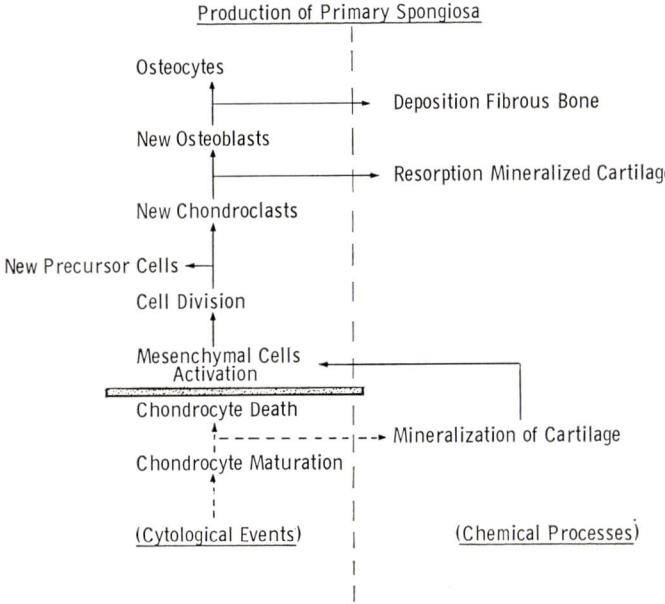

Figure 5.04. Oriented in the same manner as the previous figure with respect to the tibia shown in Figure 3.02. The horizontal shaded bar here represents the secondary spongiosa; below it (omitted here for purposes of clarity) would lie the histogenetic processes of chondrogenesis and the production of primary spongiosa diagrammed in the previous figure. Above that bar lie on the left the various cellular, and on the right the chemical events, sequences, and processes that replace the primary by the secondary (i.e. permanent) spongiosa. Temporally later events lie above earlier ones.

TABLE 5.03
DISEASES RELATED TO THE ENDOCHONDRAL OSSIFICATION SEQUENCES

ENOS Stage	Disease Arising from a Disturbance in the Step and the Change in the Step
1. Chondroblast proliferation	Gigantism (U*) Marfan's syndrome (U) Eunuchism (U) Achondroplasia (D*) Pituitary dwarf (D) Chondrodystrophies (D) (?) Rickets, malnutrition (D)
2. Cartilage matrix synthesis per cell	(?) Chondrodystrophies (D) (?) Rickets (D)
3. Calcification of cartilage matrix	Rickets of all kinds (D) Morquio's disease (D) Hurler's disease (D) Jansen's disease (D)
4. Replacement of calcified cartilage by primary spongiosa	ªOsteopetrosis (D) Scurvy (D) Plumbism (D)
5. Replacement of primary by secondary spongiosa	ᵇOsteopetrosis (D) Scurvy (D) Plumbism (D)

*U: Up; D: Down

The left column lists the five stages into which this text divides the ENOS process, while the right column lists some diseases known to associate with delays or accelerations in each stage. The numbers correspond to those in the text.

ing from studies by Gong et al,[40] spongy bone comprises approximately 20 per cent of the true mass or weight of bony tissue in the young adult skeleton but well over 50 per cent of the total bony surface exposed to osteoclasts and osteoblasts. Diseases exist, such as osteogenesis imperfecta, in which a deficient amount of spongy lamellar bone accumulates during growth, and as a consequence an adult person affected by this disease never has an adequate supply of the lamellar bone.

Diseases

Failure to replace the primary by secondary spongiosa represents the basic defect in a second and apparently the commoner

The Endochondral Ossification Process

type of osteopetrosis (based on the limited amounts of biopsy material we have seen; to my knowledge these types have not yet been reported as such in the literature).

Table 5.03 lists some diseases known to arise as defects at each step in the ENOS process.

QUESTIONS

1. In the broad scheme shown in Figure 5.01, list the general factors that can influence ENOS activity.
2. According to the scheme in Figure 1.03, list the factors that can influence ENOS activity.
3. List the basic cellular steps in ENOS; the basic chemical steps; the basic morphological steps.
4. List what we believe at present comprise the functions or purposes of ENOS; of chondrogenesis.
5. Why would study of metaphyseal activity in experimental growing animals probably shed little light on diseases peculiar to adult skeletons?
6. Why would study of STH effects on chondrocyte biochemical processes shed little light on the basic causative defect in gigantism; in achondroplasia?

Chapter VI

Biomechanical Responses of Hyaline Chondral Growth

Chondral tissues pose the general problems of finding and understanding the phenomena that regulate their creation, growth, maintenance, repair, and their structural adaptations to biomechanical needs. We also need to understand their injuries, diseases, neoplasms, and degenerative processes.

This chapter considers only one of those problems: the biomechanical response characteristics of chondral growth as those characteristics relate to speed and direction. Once identified, these characteristics find ready and wide use in clinical orthopaedics.

INTRODUCTION

While a modern physician probably memorizes no greater number of facts than did Hippocrates or his predecessors over 2,000 years ago, we today possess far greater power to alter the natural course of disease than did our ancient antecedents. Much of this gain derives from the peculiarly human trait of recording experience, in writing as well as by other means, so that it passes down through the generations of man. In the process each generation retains access to contemporaneously helpful knowledge and can discard that which has become outmoded.

However, another and quite different factor also operates in augmenting our mastery over disease, and by virtue of our present level of scientific development it offers a vastly greater potential

TABLE 6.01

ABBREVIATIONS APPEARING IN CHAPTER VI

CDH:	Congenital dysplasia of the hip
ENOS:	Endochondral ossification and/or chondral growth
ITT:	Internal tibial torsion
STH:	Growth hormone; somatotrophic hormone

for advancement in the immediate future than does a mere record of more and yet more purely empirical experience. This factor consists of the discovery of the basic *principles of action* which underlie mammalian physiology, whose aberrations produce disease. Gradually in the past and at an accelerating rate in this century we begin to discover, understand, and use these principles of action, sometimes in designing experiments, sometimes in diagnostic analyses, and occasionally even in therapeutic design (in fact, we can even use them to structure a book, something done within these pages but probably not yet obvious to the reader). Such principles allow us to proceed directly to the core of otherwise apparently bewilderingly complex problems with maximally efficient and even seemingly magical utilization of one's memory, intellectual process, and time.

This chapter formalizes in a preliminary and rough way a complex of fairly simple biomechanical principles of action which I have inferred from the spatial behavior of growing chondral complex tissues, such as articular cartilage and epiphyseal plate, and which predict and/or explain that behavior. These principles "work" in the predictive and operational senses in projecting forwards in time the effects on the speed and direction of chondral growth of various clinical treatments and equally so in designing effective new treatments. Consequently, they could serve all practitioners of the healing arts who work with the growing musculoskeletal system. In addition to allowing us to plan and achieve better therapy, these principles also promise better diagnostic depth and range which, hopefully in the near future, we may begin to tap.

A subsequent chapter will deal with somewhat analogous biomechanical principles which govern the response of fibrous tissues, and a later volume with the modeling phenomenon (i.e. "sculpting") of lamellar bone and some of the biomechanical properties of hyaline articular cartilage tissue once it has been produced. I do not discuss here another interesting problem, but because of its probable importance I will identify it here: Structures such as articular cartilage have a "grain," meaning that the collagen within it exhibits not anarchy but considerable overall order in relation to local mechanical force resultants. What factors establish that order? Since the collagen bundles arise outside the cell as polymers of the basic tropocollagen molecule, one infers some microenvironmental physical-chemical situation as being responsible, possibly the electric fields discussed by Bassett[10] and Becker.[11, 12] The collagen in organs made of fibrous tissue (such as tendon, ligament) and lamellar bone also exhibits this phenomenon, as does that in the dentine of the tooth. Clearly some kind of transducing mechanism converts mechanical stress into collagen polymer alignment at this level, and identifying it represents an important research problem for the future.

With that omission in mind, then, let us turn to the less fundamental but far more important, clinically speaking, problems of how chondral growth speed and direction relate to mechanical forces.

THE CHONDRAL MODELING LAWS

Functions of Endochondral Ossification

The responses of growing hyaline cartilage to mechanical factors (and the response of the ENOS mechanism, which depends ultimately—as previously noted—upon chondral growth) assume significance only in relation to their biomechanically oriented functions. Table 6.02 lists for review some of the basic behavioral properties of the endochondral ossification process; these represent the "strings" of the chondral "harp" played upon by biomechanical factors. Figure 6.01 locates the subject matter of this chapter in the overall scheme of skeletal organization. Keeping in mind the philosophical point that biological subsystems usually have few and simple true functions, here these first-order functions of ENOS certainly must include the following five:

1. It *adds new length* in the overall sense to growing bones, primarily under the controlling influence of endocrine factors such as somatotrophic hormone or STH and the hormones of the thyroid axis (first- and second-order functions). Other than identifying that important and basic property at this juncture, this chapter will not consider it further.

TABLE 6.02

ENDOCHONDRAL OSSIFICATION

Morphological Events	Production of new chondroblasts → production of new cartilage matrix → calcification of matrix → replacement by primary spongiosa → replacement by secondary spongiosa and marrow tissue.
Behavioral events and processes	(Mesenchymal cell activation → proliferation → differentiation of chondroblasts → secretion of chondroitin sulfates A and C plus collagen → mineralization) = chondrogenesis; → (Mesenchymal cell activation → proliferation differentiation of osteoblasts → secretion of chondroitin sulfates A and B plus collagen → mineralization); = fibrous bone; (Mesenchymal cell activation → proliferation differentiation osteoblasts → secretion chondroitin sulfates A and B plus collagen → lamellar bone → mineralization) = replacement by secondary spongiosa; → Turnover; blood-bone exchange.
Functions	Creation of new bone length and new trabecular structural mass (i.e. growth) and hematopoietic potential; establishing joint architecture and alignment; a medium compliance structural material rigid in compression, tension, and shear. A means for transferring diffused mechanical loads to concentrated regions of maximal rigidity and minimum compliance. A means of healing fractures.

When biomechanical factors act on growing cartilaginous regions of bone to modify its architecture, they do so by means of one or more of the activities listed here.

2. *It determines the shapes and sizes of growing articulations,* in such a way as to permit mechanically unrestricted joint motion only around those axes determined by the anatomy of muscles and the neural integration of their contractural activity, as well as by certain factors which operate during embryological development and which have accomplished their purpose and become inoperative by and after the third month of gestation (third-order functions). I conceive this function as arising by producing regionally localized modifications of the overall speed of growth in length; thus, by exerting a holding action here and allowing growth to proceed optimally there, one can produce quite com-

124 The Physiology of Cartilaginous, Fibrous, and Bony Tissue

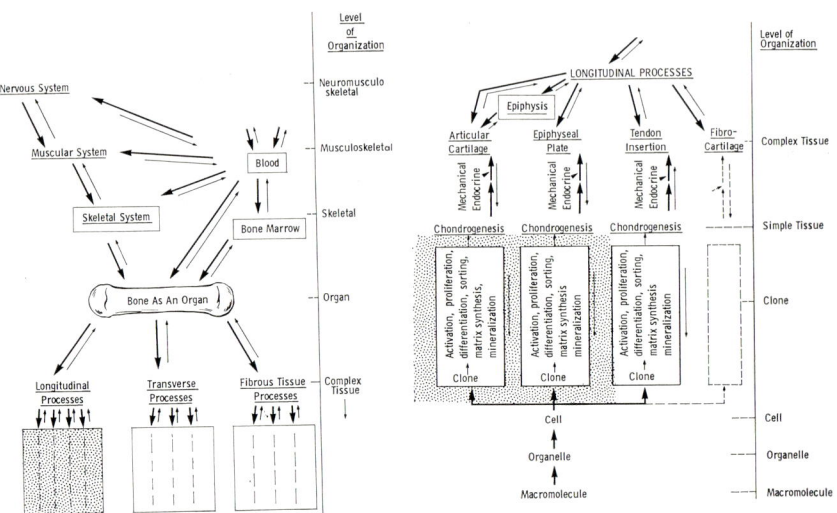

Figure 6.01. The stippled zones locate the subject matter of this chapter in the overall scheme of skeletal organization. It deals with the longitudinally acting class of cellular subsystems involved in skeletal physiology, and with only two categories of those (see right side).

plicated shapes. We can write this as a word diagram, worth the effort because of its great importance to clinical medicine:

$$
\begin{array}{ccc}
(Chondrogenetic\ growth\ potential) & \rightleftarrows & (Endocrine\ regulation) \\
\downarrow & & \downarrow \\
Random\ growth & & Coordinated\ growth \\
& & \downarrow \\
(Control\ of\ architecture) & \rightarrow & (Biomechanical\ regulation)
\end{array}
$$

This and the next function comprise the main subjects of this chapter.

3. ENOS *establishes and maintains the alignment* of various joints during growth and thus of adjacent articulating bones with respect to each other. This represents one consequence of the second function just described, and it, too, occurs primarily under the controlling influence of muscular forces, including the particular features of their anatomical location and orientation, their contractural timing, and relative magnitudes, dictated by neurocybernetic factors extrinsic to the ENOS mechanism.

4. The ENOS process *forms the major fraction of the trabecular bone* in the skeleton, a matter returned to in Volume III.

5. *It moves bony attachments of fibrous tissue structures during growth* (i.e. tendons, ligaments, and sheets of fascia), in such a way that they maintain their relative or proportional locations on a bone's surfaces even though this requires several centimeters of motion in tissue space to do so, as the bone increases in size more than a hundred-fold during its total growth.

Chrondral Biomechanical Response Characteristics

Having specified five first-order biomechanical functions of ENOS in terms of the body generally, we can next state in a simple and modernized form the principle recognized as the Heuter-Volkmann law. To those who have made previous but possibly partially unsuccessful attempts to travel the logical route that begins in the next paragraph and ends at the conclusion of the next chapter, I urge patience; in the operational sense (exactly the sense in which I offer this material for your use) the model outlined here remains internally consistent in clinical use, meaning it does not predict things contrary to what really happen. This model will receive the cognomen "The Chondral Modeling Laws." It has two parts: one consisting of the Heuter-Volkmann principle, the other of a group of six additional principles which I formulated.

Heuter-Volkmann Principle

1. *The chondral growth rate decreases under excessive compression force.*

To that basic law we must add my own corollaries—without which it does not work properly—as follows:

2. The growth rate-mechanical force response characteristic exhibits *a biphasic curve.* Henceforth, we will signify the curve that represents it as the *growth/force-response characteristic.*

3. In the pathological range, increasing compression force perpendicular to a chondral growth plane progressively retards

growth; within the physiologic range, increasing compression accelerates it.

4. Within the physiologic mechanical force range of magnitudes, chondral growth speed in a region under compression exceeds that in one under tension.

5. Within the physiological range of mechanical force magnitudes, overall chondral growth direction parallels the time-averaged resultant of the local mechanical compression and/or tension forces.

> *Note:* We now have elementary rules that can serve to predict both chondral growth *speed* and *direction* under given circumstances. Shortly we will look at them in action more closely. First, for future reference, Table 6.03 summarizes the above rules; second, we must next describe a few ancillary properties displayed by actual, living skeletons.

6. *Qualifications:* As with any other principle of action, these rules focus better in the light of their peculiar behavioral properties and exclusions found under specific conditions. Some qualifications of major concern receive attention now, and following that the text will discuss a few clinically pertinent but very general examples of these principles in action. The subsequent chapter will then apply them to a few illustrative clinical problems.

The Time-averaging Property: The rate and direction of growth of an endochondral plate respond somehow to the *time-averaged resultant* of the tension and compression forces acting across it. The duration of that averaging period (in the terminology we will

TABLE 6.03

CHONDRAL MODELING LAWS

1. Chondral growth decreases under excessive compression force.
2. The chondral growth/force-response characteristic exhibits a biphasic curve.
3. In the physiologic range, chondral growth *speed* in compression exceeds that in tension.
4. In the physiologic range, local chondral growth *direction* parallels the time-averaged local force resultant.
5. This system averages mechanical resultants over time.

use in Volume III, "sigma for chondral modeling") approximates the time the system takes to respond and successfully adapt to a change in its typical mechanical loads, and it increases with aging. An approximate order of time for infants would equal three months; by maturity at age 15-18 years it has become infinite for practical purposes. Because of the averaging property, a mild but constant load could easily exert more total effect on chondral growth than very large but brief and seldomly applied forces.

The Physiologic Range: A "physiologic range" of forces across chondral growth planes exists, meaning amounts of compression and/or tension which fall within a normal rather than a pathological range. That physiologic range extends from some limit of tension over to zero and then farther over to some physiologic limit of compression (on the order of magnitude of 50-100 lbs/in^2).

The "physiologic range" of forces probably spans extremes separated by more than 300 pounds per square inch. Within this physiologic range, relatively small but nevertheless very important changes in growth rate follow changes in the average amount and/or type of force (i.e. whether tension or compression) applied across the plate. However, when a compression load exceeds that physiologic limit, large disturbances can ensue, usually as an obvious decrease in growth rate which, with even further increase in the compression load, can lead to total arrest of further growth. This latter behavioral property underlies therapeutic epiphyseodesis by stapling or bone grafting, means we often employ to equalize limb length discrepancies during growth.

The response of the endochondral growth rate to tension and compression forces follows approximately the curve shown in Figure 6.02, henceforth termed the "growth/force-response characteristic"; this constitutes one of the most important items of new information of clinical utility in this book. Experimental and quantitative definition and validation of this curve, with respect to its shape, its slopes, and the absolute magnitudes of the values on its axes, remain undone but constitute an extremely important and potentially very productive area for future biomechanical, clinically oriented research.

128   *The Physiology of Cartilaginous, Fibrous, and Bony Tissue*

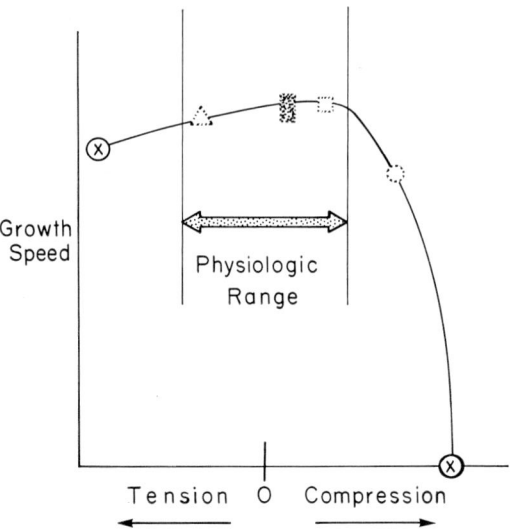

Figure 6.02. This curve, published for the first time here, relates the responses of the speed of chondral growth to mechanical tension and compression forces. As the flexure-drift laws represent a significant breakthrough in understanding the mechanical and architectural principles guiding modeling of lamellar bone, this represents a similar advance in understanding the mechanical and architectural principles guiding modeling of growing cartilage. The vertical axis represents chondral growth speed according to some arbitrary scale of absolute units (such as millimeters per year). The horizontal axis represents tension and compression forces as an infinitely variable continuum, ranging from maximum tension on the left through zero at the center, and into the compression range on the right. This curve applies only to forces aligned perpendicularly to the direction of chondral growth, and to the *time-averaged resultants of such forces,* not to occasional or momentary ones.

Shearing Phenomena: Cartilaginous growth planes of relatively normal physiologic and mechanical properties seem to exhibit trivial responses in growth *rate* to shearing loads, whether those exist in the presence of superimposed compression or tension loads. With regard to *direction* of growth under combined but physiologic-magnitude compression-shearing and tension-shearing force couples, Figure 6.03 diagrams the fact that they yield gradually to the shearing component; it effectively realigns the net

Biomechanical Responses of Hyaline Chondral Growth

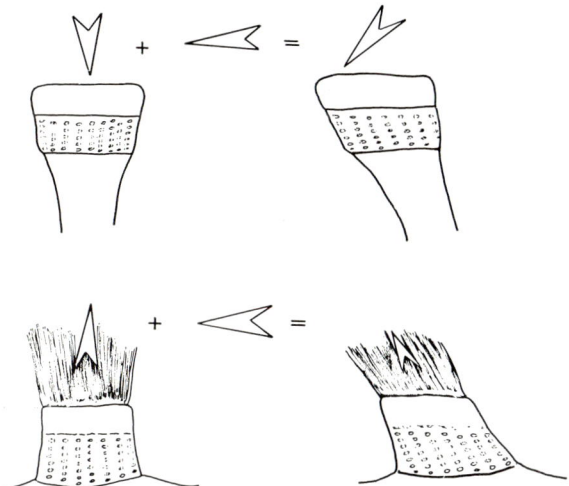

Figure 6.03. Top: When to a compression load acting perpendicularly across a chondral growth plane, such as an epiphyseal plate (left), one adds a net shearing force distributed evenly over the whole plate, that makes the chondral growth plane move or creep or grow slowly sideways in the direction of the shearing force and without developing any tilt or change in the vertical direction of growth of the whole plane relative to its original alignment in space. The arrows show the individual forces and (right) their resultant.

Bottom: When to a tension load acting perpendicularly across a chondral growth plane, such as a tendon attachment to bone, one adds a shearing force (as for example by pulling sideways instead of perpendicularly to bone surface), again the growth plane moves slowly sideways, again in the direction of the shearing force, and again without tilting.

direction of growth normal to the shear. No real tilt arises in the anatomical orientation of the plane as it does this.

Now let us examine several rather general consequences of these principles in action.

General Situations of the Laws in Action

1. Three general cases of major clinical concern and illustrative value exist: the *rectangular epiphysis*, the *ball-socket* configuration, and the *local articular incongruity*. They convey sufficient

grasp of chondral growth responses to biomechanical factors that the clinically oriented reader should study and assimilate them before proceeding any further in this volume. First, note the following features, readily apparent clinically when you look for them in the response of any chondral growth plane to mechanical factors:

Speed: A unilateral and random increase in the speed of growth across any chondral growth plane will predictably change the alignment of the associated joint, as shown in Figure 6.04. By altering the alignment of muscle forces and gravity acting across the joint, this tends to concentrate on the right-hand side more than its normal share of the compression loads carried across the joint. *When within the physiologic range of force magnitude,* for example, as might arise by virtue of the purely random variations which characterize all biological processes, growth speed on that side then will *increase* slightly because the response characteristic has moved slightly to the right (from the dotted rectangle to the dotted open square region on the curve in Figure 6.02). That increase then corrects the malalignment. Thus, an extremely important property of the system we discuss is as follows:

Small random errors in joint and limb alignment evoke a negative feedback mode of response, one which subsequently corrects them.

This occurs because the growth rate on the *slightly* overloaded right side speeds up somewhat because of that small overload, and that speedup acts to correct the malalignment. If true, this means the following: *During growth, normal joints should tend to align perpendicularly to the resultant of all the mechanical compression forces they carry.* Since muscular forces easily exceed those of gravity, joint alignment should obey directly the spatial dictates of muscular anatomy and functional patterns more than that of the pull of gravity. As a matter of interest, they do.

If joint angulation or malalignment become excessive (as occurs occasionally following trauma or polio, in spastic cerebral palsy, or even rarely during "normal" growth), so that the compression load on the right side increases to a point on the descending limb of the curve (the region of the dotted open circle) in Figure 6.02,

Biomechanical Responses of Hyaline Chondral Growth 131

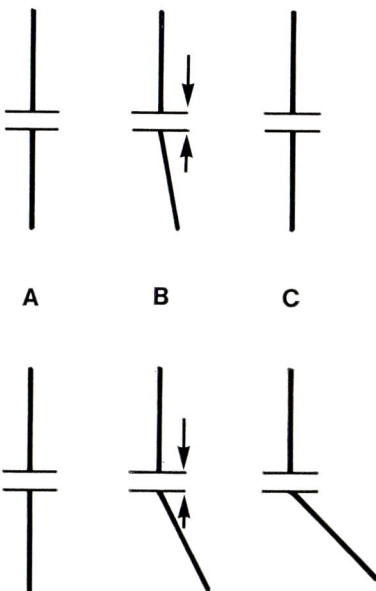

Figure 6.04. Top, A: Diagram of a normally aligned knee as seen from the front. If random variations accelerated growth on the left side, then the alignment of the joint would change to *B*, thereby increasing modestly the time-averaged amount of compression on its right, as shown in *C*. That changes the local growth rate to correspond to the region shown by the dotted open square in Figure 6.02, leading to increased subsequent growth speed. Simultaneously, the other side of the plate moves over in its rate/force-response characteristic to the region of the dotted open triangle in Figure 6.02, which decreases its growth. These two changes act to reestablish the previous normal alignment of the joint. The above behavior typifies that of any *negative feedback system*. In this one, the "error" detected by the system represents unequal force distribution (which the malalignment causes); the feedback loop constitutes the compression forces, and the manner in which they affect the growth rate establishes the response as conforming to the negative feedback mode. *Bottom:* Should the malalignment become pathological in degree as in *E*, the growth force-response characteristic moves even farther over into the descending limb of the curve, the region of the dotted open circle on the right hand part of the curve in Figure 6.02. That now *decreases* growth speed on the right relative to the left side and leads to subsequent increase in deformity, which further compresses the right side, and so on. In other words, the system now behaves in the *positive feedback mode* or as a "vicious cycle."

132 *The Physiology of Cartilaginous, Fibrous, and Bony Tissue*

subsequent chondral growth on that side falls behind that of the other side so that further growth makes the situation worse. This then has now converted to a *positive feedback* or "vicious cycle" mode of response.

Direction: As to the overall direction of growth of a chondral growth plane, Figures 6.04 and 6.05 illustrate the observed facts. Adding shear across a plane of endochondral growth tends to make the epiphysis slip sideways in the direction of the shearing component, although so slowly in life (see the x-rays of the knee in Fig. 6.06) as to represent a form of mechanical creep analogous to that which occrs in many man-made structural materials. When

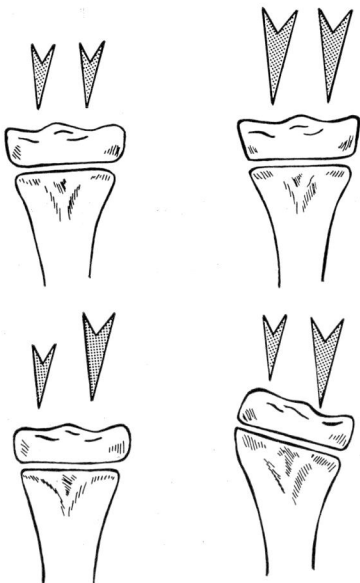

Figure 6.05. At the upper left, the proximal tibial epiphysis as seen from the front carries compression loads whose time-averaged resultants represent the dark arrows. When equal bilaterally, the subsequent growth pattern conforms to the situation at A and B. When the resultants on each side become sufficiently unequal (in terms of loads per unit area sustaining it) as at C, so as to load one side into the descending limb (i.e. the right side) of the growth/force-response characteristic curve of Figure 6.02, then the situation at D develops. If a shearing force were added equally to both sides, some gradual sideways slippage would occur, as in the next figure.

Biomechanical Responses of Hyaline Chondral Growth 133

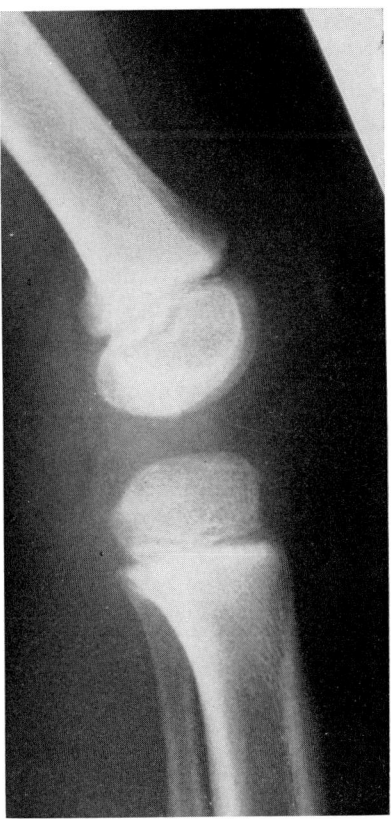

Figure 6.06. Lateral x-ray of the knee of a skeletally normal child. Note that as the knee extends *during the weight-bearing phase* of walking and running, the femoral and tibial condyles move on each other in such a way as to create a drag or shearing force on each respective epiphyseal plate. This force pushes the tibial plate *rearwards,* in real life causing it to slip slowly that way during growth. While the reaction to that drag acting on the femoral plate should tend to slip it forwards, another factor arises there which does not affect the tibia: The patella, due to quadriceps muscle tension, pushes it rearwards, too, and far more effectively than the frictional drag of the joint pushes it forwards; as a result it, too, slips gradually rearwards during growth. While an oppositely acting shearing force arises during the knee flexion occurring in the swing phase of gait, no weight and consequently greatly reduced muscle forces exist then, so the frictional "drag" of that motion does not equal in magnitude (and so cancel out) that of the opposite one. A similar phenomenon explains why, in the idiopathic epiphyseolisthesis of the capital femoral epiphysis that occurs about age 12, the epiphysis always displaces posteriorly on the underlying femoral neck.

the mechanical properties of the cartilage become abnormal, such creep can cause significant and pathological amounts of slippage of epiphyseal plates, which appears for example in various kinds of rickets, in capital femoral epiphyseolisthesis of adolescence, and possibly, as Dr. L. Z. Shifrin and C. Shock suggest, in the rotatory spinal deformity usually arising in idiopathic scoliosis.

2. *Rectangular vs. ball-socket epiphyses:* In life, the speed and direction rules already stated act in two geometrically different situations which lead apparently to two grossly different response characteristics. (These responses are not as dissimilar as they may seem at first glance but we need not write that story here.)

To review briefly the case of the *rectangular epiphysis,* any malalignment between the orientations of the growth plane and the time-averaged load resultant lying within the physiological range of Figure 6.02 causes the plate to realign itself perpendicular to the resultant of the compression loads it carries. Usually that resultant will pass directly through the middle of the plate. Given normal mechanical properties, it may also displace laterally in the direction of shear when affected by a compression-shear couple, as in Figures 6.03 and 6.05. It will angulate progressively in response to any pathological-range increase of compression on one side (i.e. moving to the descending limb of the curve in Figure 6.02), owing to decreased growth speed on that side, as shown in Figure 6.05. The worse the angulation, the greater the growth retardation on that side, which leads to yet more angulation with further growth. I suspect such a situation exists in Blount's disease, based in part upon how well the situation has responded (in my own experience plus that of C. L. Mitchell, D. C. Mitchell, and E. R. Guise, which may not agree with that of others) to effective and early correction by open valgus osteotomy.

3. For the case of the *ball-socket* configuration, and concentrating on the ball for the moment, another factor contributes to the above response pattern. To understand it, note that unequal thicknesses of spongy bone lie between the time-averaged resultant of the abnormally aligned compression load in Figure 6.07B and the underlying regions of the epiphyseal plate. In other words, the ball does not receive that resultant distributed evenly over its

Biomechanical Responses of Hyaline Chondral Growth

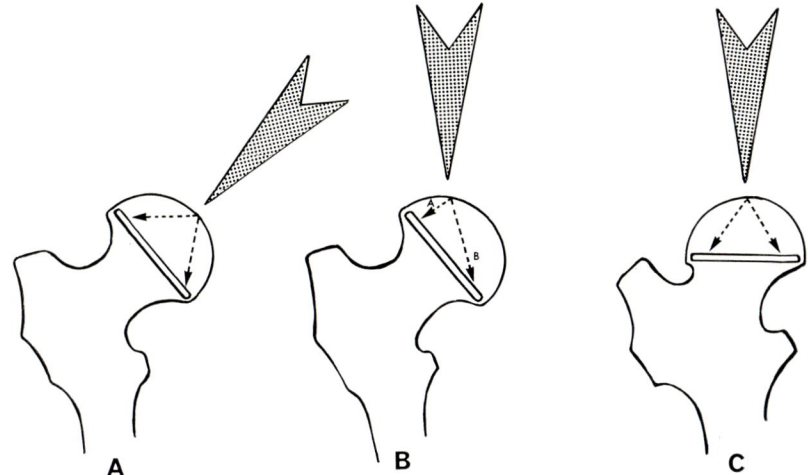

Figure 6.07. Normally, in a ball-and-socket joint the epiphyseal plate of the ball aligns perpendicularly to the time-averaged mechanical force resultant acting across the joint *(A)*. Should extrinsic factors (such as obturator-abductor paralysis) change the alignment of that resultant towards the vertical, as in *B*, the springy or compliant quality of the spongiosa over the plate plus greatly differing thicknesses of it cause the loading on the left side of the plate to increase relative to the other, loading that region into the decending limb of the curve in Figure 6.02. This invokes a retardation in chondral growth speed which acts in the negative feedback mode, as shown in *C*. Only when the change in alignment of the resultant occurs too late (age +10 years) will this not occur, for thereafter insufficient growth potential remains to allow reorientation of the plate by such means.

whole surface; rather, it peaks at one region as shown. The bone interposed between plate and joint has a "springy" quality; technically, it exhibits *compliance* or "give" rather than perfect rigidity, and thicker layers of spongy bone provide more total give than thin ones. As a consequence, the part of the plate nearest the source of that force (i.e. its left side) carries enough more compression load to retard chondral growth speed relative to that on the right side, which the greater overlying thickness of springy cancellous bone "padding" somewhat protects from that load. The resulting faster growth on the right than on the left subsequently realigns the plate until it achieves the state shown in

6.07E. There it again lies perpendicular to the resultant of all the time-averaged compression loads carried by the ball, and thereafter it retains that orientation unless the load resultant should change again.

This, then, illustrates again a negative feedback mode of response. These response characteristics of rectangular and ball-and-socket epiphyses give rise to a clinically useful operational rule describing the effects on growth direction of mechanical forces lying within the physiologic range, as follows:

The plane of the epiphyseal plate (note—not of the articular cartilage) of rectangular and ball-shaped epiphyses aligns perpendicularly to the time-averaged resultant of the compression forces they carry.

Ball configurations would include the femoral capital and proximal humeral epiphyseal plates and all metatarsal and metacarpal heads.

4. *The Local Incongruity:* This case illustrates some effects of the chondral modeling laws on growing *articular cartilage;* they act more (but not exclusively) to determine the *shape* of the joint, where the epiphyseal plate responses act more (but again not exclusively) to determine its overall *alignment.* This happens because the articular cartilage lies directly exposed to incongruities and so readily becomes loaded over into the descending limb of the response-characteristics curve in Figure 6.02, where in the same joint a thick mass of epiphyseal spongiosa tends to shield the epiphyseal plate from such effects. In effect *this difference causes the articular chondral growth to respond sensitively to the geometry of the joint surfaces, while the epiphyseal plate responds more sensitively to the overall alignment of the joint.*

Consider thus Figure 6.08 which illustrates an ankle as seen from the front. At *A*, the normal sideways or laterally acting loads applied to a foot during an active day dissipate at the subtalar joint, thereby protecting the ankle joint from those forces. If, as in *B*, subtalar ankylosis arose early in childhood, then the lateral forces just referred to would affect the ankle joint. Note that pushing the foot towards your left (as in *B*) causes the corners of the talus to become a local incongruity exerting large unit compres-

Biomechanical Responses of Hyaline Chondral Growth 137

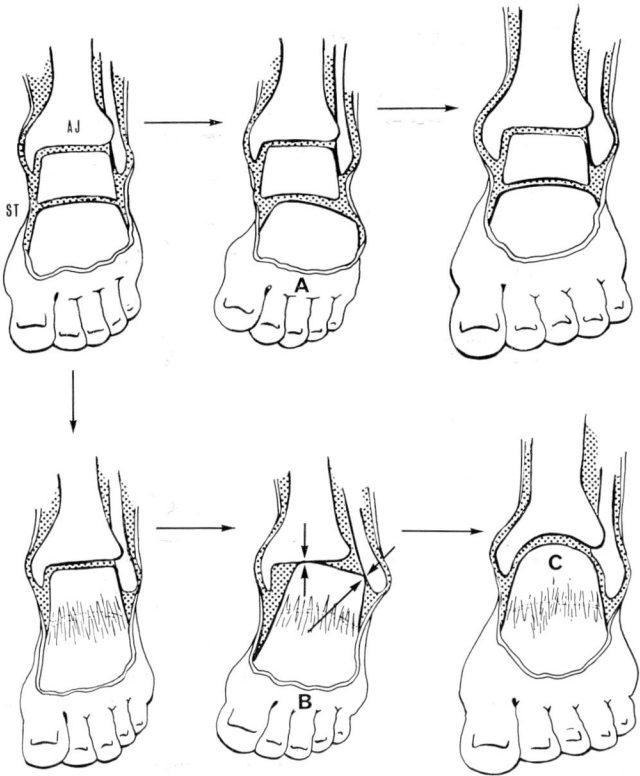

Figure 6.08. Top: On the left we see an ankle diagrammed as seen from the front. The subtalar joint (ST) absorbs the sideways "whip" or rotatory motion to which normal daily use subjects all ankles and feet. If, as in the bottom diagram, some mechanical limitation arises in childhood which limits that motion, then the corners of the talus experience large compression loads as indicated in the middle. This leads to decreased local chondral growth (note: now of articular cartilage rather than of epiphyseal plate), so that the growing structure modifies its shape, progressing in time to a ball-and-socket ankle joint, bottom right.

sion forces on the impinging regions, which represent a small area of the total cartilaginous surface of the joint. Locally, these large forces move the chondral growth/force-response characteristic towards the descending limb (dotted open circle region) of the response curve shown in Figure 6.02. Thus, growth in the im-

138   *The Physiology of Cartilaginous, Fibrous, and Bony Tissue*

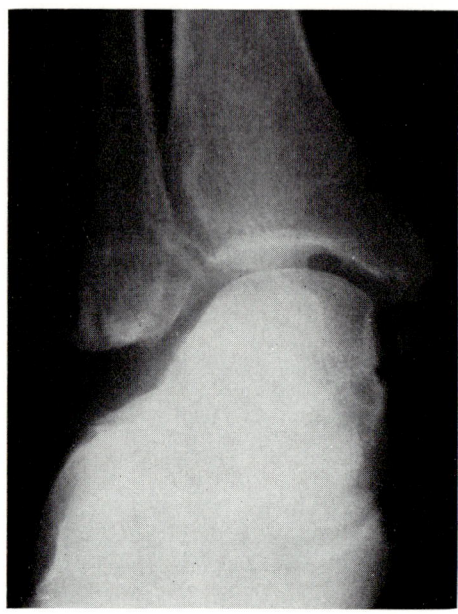

Figure 6.09. An AP x-ray of the ankle of a 50-year-old patient who has had absent subtalar motion since early childhood. The chondral growth/force response characteristic described in the text led to the development of a true ball-and-socket ankle joint. This phenomenon, not common but long known, supports the proposal made later in this book that the muscle forces acting in intrauterine life and during infancy determine in large part the gross architectural features of joints.

pinging regions slows down relative to the other regions. Over time this leads to the ball configuration at *C*.

Finally, Figure 6.09 shows an actual example of this phenomenon in a patient of Dr. Wallace Johnson's. In this instance, the condition known as the "ball-and-socket ankle joint" arose bilaterally because of a congenital synostosis across that subtalar joint.

   Nota bene: Function determines structure.

Having described the relatively simple and basic elements of the chondral growth/force-response characteristics, the next chapter will examine some clinical problems to which the Heuter-Volkmann relations apply and which explain why conventional treatments have worked well and dependably, although they evolved purely by an empirical, trial-and-error process rather than from any rational exploitation of this law.

QUESTIONS

1. Why does the femoral head initially always drift *backwards* on the neck in slipped capital femoral epiphysis of young adolescents?
2. What (according to this text) most directly determines the shape of a joint, and what determines its alignment?
3. List the chondral growth/force-response characteristics.
4. Where do these characteristics fit into the overall scheme of skeletal physiology?
5. What roles does this chapter relegate to any genetic factors that participate in determining joint architecture; limb alignment?

Chapter VII

Clinical Application of the Chondral Modeling Laws

The Chondral Modeling Laws can explain major aspects of both the genesis and the effects of treatment of congenital dislocation of the hip, internal tibial torsion, club foot, metatarsus varus, and allied deformities, as well as the normal architectural configuration and alignment of most joints.

CONGENITAL HIP DYSPLASIA

In this and the following analyses we tackle problems that have long concerned orthopaedists, which have long resisted successful analysis (or at least analysis consistent with known facts) relative to their causes, and which have engendered some controversy in that regard. Thus, some who read these paragraphs and who find within them unfamiliar views may react negatively towards them. To the students of such individuals I offer this: Whether ultimately the rationale supporting it crumbles before the onslaught of future research or not, *applying that rationale has worked consistently*, for resident and attending alike, in my clinical practice for well over 15 years without yet exposing any major flaw in its construction or operation. Paraphrased, it succeeds in the operational sense. Thus, one may take the trouble to learn this material in confidence that it will work for him, too, in clinical applications. Obviously, I would not publish this material were I even faintly dubious as to its validity.

TABLE 7.01

ABBREVIATIONS APPEARING IN CHAPTER VII

CDH:	Congenital dysplasia of the hip
ITT:	Internal tibial torsion

Clinical Application of the Chondral Modeling Laws 141

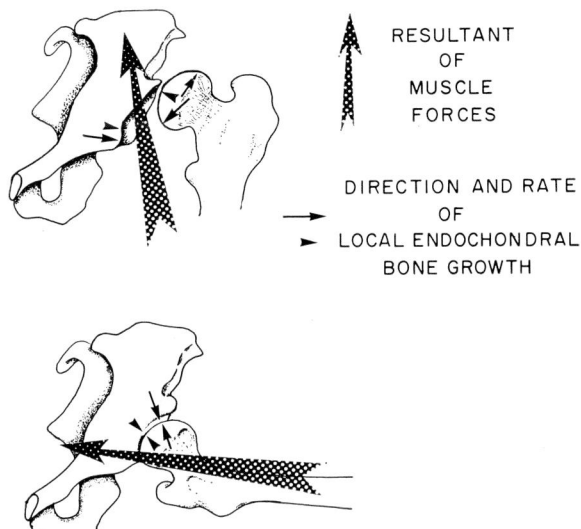

Figure 7.1. Top: The situation the author proposes represents the essential elements of the usual (but not all) congenital hip dislocation, which begins in infancy as "dysplasia" and can be diagnosed as Stanisavljevic has described.[89] It gradually progresses to the stage shown here at approximately nine to twelve months of age, and if untreated will then progress to frank dislocation. The elements of this situation include an abnormally vertical resultant of all the muscle forces acting across the hip, thereby concentrating mechanical force on the superoposterior margin of the socket, which decreases subsequent growth there relative to lateralwards growth of the socket's medial wall, thus leading to progressive subluxation and eventually dislocation. *Bottom:* Holding the hip abducted by any means (such as a splint or cast) realigns the muscle forces relative to the acetabulum so that all now pull the head against its medial wall and relieve the upper-posterior margin. This reverses the previous pattern of growth and so acts to correct the problem.

Figure 7.01 diagrams the common predislocation situation as we usually find it when this problem becomes recognized clinically (for good reviews, see Stanisavljevic,[89, 90]). For our needs the essential facts of this situation constitute impingement of the femoral head against the superoposterior margin of the cartilaginous acetabulum; this concentrates the compression loads which normally lie evenly distributed over the whole femoral head (and which in infants represent muscular forces primarily) onto the relatively small impinging regions of both the acetabulum and the femoral head. This concentration overloads this impinging region in compression, shifts the local growth/force-response characteristic over towards the descending limb of the curve in Figure 6.02, and so retards subsequent local chondral growth. Simultaneously, chondral growth can proceed near its optimal pace in the medial regions of the ball-socket joint surfaces, since the above impingement substantially relieved them of such loads (even though the growth rate there should decrease slightly, that in the impinging region decreases greatly so the former exceeds the latter by a respectable amount). As a consequence of these two factors the medial wall of the acetabulum should grow laterally faster than its superior wall grows downwards, a pattern of growth which must increase further the shallowness and steepness of the socket. The latter development must further accentuate concentration of the compression forces on the acetabular rim, which further retards chondral growth there, and so on. In other words, once the local loading situation has passed out of the physiologic into the pathologic range shown in Figure 6.02, the growth/force-response characteristic converts to the positive feedback mode. Note that we do not discuss here the effects on the epiphyseal plate, which does not yet exist at this age in this joint; rather we discuss that chondral growth which occurs only a few millimeters under the articular surfaces of the head and socket, and which does so at all diarthroidial joints during growth. This illustrates a particular case of the local articular incongruity described in the previous chapter.

As diagrammed in Figure 7.01, the above changes should promote progressive lateral and posterior subluxation of the hip joint in response to the cephalad and vertically aligned pulls of the hamstrings, long adductors, rectus femoris, and psoas muscles. Interestingly, observation by numerous anatomists and clinicians reveals that exactly this can and does occur (see the monograph by Stanisavljevic.[89]).

The usual and nearly universally effective treatment for this condition in infancy consists simply of placing the thighs out in

Clinical Application of the Chondral Modeling Laws   143

full abduction, i.e. in the frog-leg position. The position itself, not the particular device used to achieve it, constitutes the essential therapeutic measure. In that attitude, the large muscles which formerly generated vertically aligned compression forces across the hip joint now act to force the femoral head medially, directly against the medial wall of the acetabulum. Simultaneously, that position relieves the superoposterior segment of the acetabulum and the region of the head originally against it, of the previously localized concentration of compression force. According to the Chondral Modeling Laws, this therapeutic (but temporary) realignment of muscle forces should now retard chondral growth of the medial parts, while allowing resumption of an optimal pace of growth by the superior parts of the joint. Both changes would act to deepen the socket and to decrease its upwards radiographic inclination. Observation verifies this also.

The Growth Rate Dependency Rules

The actual time required to attain a satisfactory depth of socket by the above means should correlate directly with the rate of chondral growth of the local parts, if I have accurately identified the underlying principles; that is, correction should occur fastest when the local growth is fastest (expressed in normalized or relative terms, such as the period of time required at that growth speed to double the diameter of the head) and slowest when no growth remains to respond to such factors. This *normalized growth rate varies* inversely with the child's age and becomes zero for practical purposes around age 15 to 18 years. Accordingly, in response to any such mode of treatment, young infants (i.e. $\approx$ 12 months) should deepen their hip sockets more quickly than older ones ($\approx$ 12 months to 36 months), and little clinically useful deepening by this mechanism should be possible after age six to eight years.

Clinical experience certainly verifies this behavioral prediction. Let us paraphrase out of that two clinically and directly useful rules of thumb, as follows:

1. *The relative and absolute endochondral growth rates con-*

stitute the chief factors determining how quickly one can correct deformities by modifying chondral growth speed patterns.

2. The total amount of growth remaining in a part determines how much total correction one may achieve by such means.

For practical clinical purposes, both of the above factors have reached zero by age 12 to 14 years.

The above reasoning strongly suggests that the primary underlying cause of CDH probably consists of an imbalance of muscular forces acting across the hip joint in early infancy, one such that the vertically aligned forces (comprising the pulls of the iliopsoas, hamstrings, *long* adductors, and rectus femoris muscles) exceed in the relative sense the more medially aligned ones crossing it (and representing chiefly the pulls of the obturator and gemelli muscles, the pyriformis, gluteus medius and minimus, tensor fascia femoris, and *short* adductors, including pectineus). Recall that during the age range in which CDH arises, the rapidly maturing pattern of synaptic connections in the spinal cord could easily vary enough to cause such an abnormal muscle contractural pattern, which one would expect to prove temporary rather than permanent. Exactly such could account for Stanisavljevic's hip-knee-hip motor strength sign.[89]

That such an imbalance could cause CDH does not by any means form a new idea, but here I propose that we now take it much more seriously than we have in the past. That idea certainly explains the high frequency of hip dislocation in cultures where the lower limbs of infants are bound together from birth, and its low frequency in cultures where babies wear voluminous diapers or ride their mother with lower limbs straddling her body. And it is not incompatible with the hunch of Dr. Wm. Smith of Ann Arbor that some abnormality of maternal hormonal patterns affects the physical properties of the hip cartilage, thereby adding another factor to the pathogenesis of CDH.

ALIGNMENT OF THE CAPITAL FEMORAL EPIPHYSIS

Another example of the Chondral Modeling Laws appears in the orientation of the plane of the capital femoral epiphyseal plate, which as previously described aligns perpendicularly to the resultant of all the compression forces acting across the hip. We described earlier the response characteristics that engender this property. Turning that relationship "upside down" (the mathematician would say *inverting* it) means that a perpendicular erected to the plane of the capital femoral epiphyseal plate in any child's hip x-ray should parallel this resultant. The x-ray in Figure 7.02 reveals a normal hip at upper left, and at the upper right the situation in a child with spastic cerebral palsy in whom the longitudinally aligned muscles of the limb (the long adductors, rectus femoris, and hamstrings) greatly overpowered the medially aligned muscles (consisting of the obturators, abductors, and short adductors). The lower left situation presented in a patient of Dr. G. Manson (of our Department of Pediatrics), in whom muscular dystrophy greatly reduced all motor power relative to body weight, leading to a more vertical alignment of the resultant.

The Analytical Inversion Rule

In dealing with clinical situations an analytical artifice can often help to identify the mechanical force abnormalities that cause a given growth-related problem. The artifice consists simply of reasoning backwards from the deformity by means of the Chondral Modeling Laws (as well as the stretch-hypertrophy and flexure-drift laws, which will come up later). As a concrete example, a given radial epiphyseal plate had angulated far too much ulnarwards during early growth in a young girl patient of mine with Ehrenfried's disease (see Fig. 7.03). A radial osteotomy was planned to correct the cosmetically objectionable ulnar deviation. The spatial orientation of the radial epiphyseal plate suggested some abnormally large compression force existed on its ulnar side, one not of muscular origin because direct examination of the power of the individual muscles with that possibility in mind revealed the ulnar carpal motors *weaker* than the radial ones, not stronger. This led me to infer some kind of "tether" joining carpus to ulna, one which did not grow as fast as the bones and so added a growth-retarding force on the lateral region of the plate.

146 *The Physiology of Cartilaginous, Fibrous, and Bony Tissue*

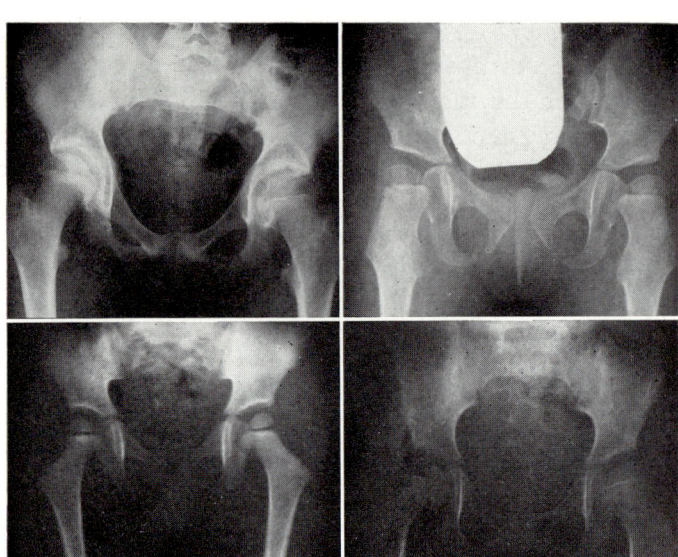

Figure 7.02. Upper left: AP x-ray of the hips of a skeletally normal child. The author proposes that a perpendicular erected to the capital epiphyseal plates parallels the *time-averaged* mechanical load resultant across the joint. Note that the metaphyseal trabeculae also parallel that resultant, and exactly so. *Lower left:* Similar x-ray of a child with pseudohypertrophic muscular dystrophy. Marked weakness of the muscles pulling medially across the hip has caused body weight to become the major load on the joint. Since it acts vertically, the capital plates have aligned themselves perpendicularly to it, i.e. parallel to the floor. *Upper right:* Severe bilateral lower-limb spasticity of that pattern characterized by overactive adductors, psoas and hamstrings, and underactive abductors and obturators. The resulting pathological **vertical** resultant of the time-averaged loads has caused the plates to align parallel to the floor. One of these hips subsequently dislocated and was corrected (as described in Volume I of this series) by rebalancing the hip motors surgically. *Lower right:* To prove that spasticity alone was not the cause of the situation shown above, here is another child with severe bilateral lower limb spasticity *but of a different pattern.* Her abductors and anatomical internal rotators were overactive and her adductors normal or slightly underactive, so she had a surplus of medially pulling muscle forces. Her capital epiphyseal plates have a normal, or possibly even supernormal, inclination away from horizontal.

Clinical Application of the Chondral Modeling Laws 147

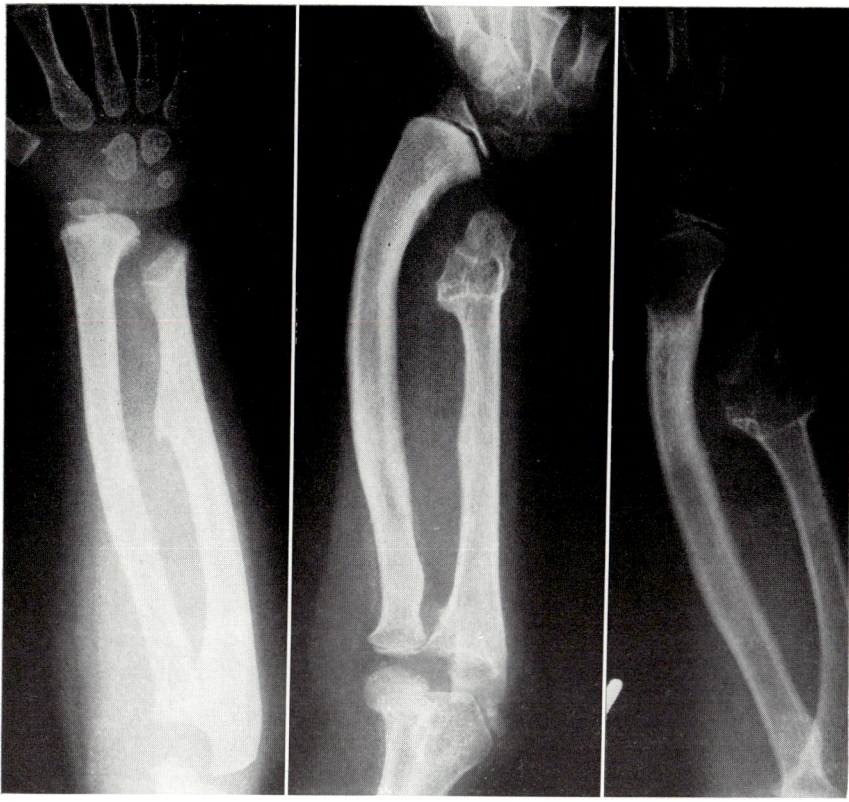

Figure 7.03. Left: A patient of mine, a young girl with hereditary multiple exostoses, x-rayed in infancy because of cartilaginous masses presenting at the wrist. Radiographically, the overall architecture appears satisfactory. *Middle:* Some six years later, more radial than ulnar longitudinal growth has created a situation in which the carpus must soon dislocate proximally and ulnarwards. *Right:* Some nine months later and after corrective cuneiform radial osteotomy. An essential step in this correction was recognition that some kind of tether had to connect distal ulna to carpus and retard longitudinal growth on that side. The first incision at operation was made in search of such a tether, and a large one was found and cut. Note the increased distance between ulna and carpus postoperatively, compared to the preoperative situation in the middle.

The Chondral Growth Laws work in clinical practice!

At surgery exactly such a tether of thick fibrous tissue was found on both wrists, and the correction of the overall deformity illustrated on the right could not possibly have been achieved without releasing it, unless I had shortened the radius by nearly 2 cm, an undesirable choice since the child's forearms were already shorter than normal.

INTERNAL TIBIAL TORSION (ITT)

A third example of the Chondral Modeling Laws appears in treating internal tibial torsion (ITT) in young children with splints holding the feet turned outwards. At nine to twelve months of age such therapy can correct completely 45 degrees of ITT within only four to five months (not all of these correct themselves if left alone, contrary to the statements of some authorities, as Dr. Joseph Hohl of this department can attest). This correction does not occur in the true bony part of the tibia for, as F. Gaynor Evans and D. Enlow would observe, this, like chalk, possesses such rigidity that it will break rather than deform plastically in response to any applied torque. The actual correction of the ITT occurs in the cartilaginous regions at the ankle and knee joints, which contain several chondral growth planes (both epiphyseal and subarticular) which respond in the previously described manner to the altered locations, concentrations, and orientations of the compression forces crossing them which the external rotation splint causes. Figure 7.04 illustrates what occurs in the knee, where I believe approximately 75 percent of the grossly visible correction of ITT usually arises.

To understand that figure and all analogous problems in all other joints, remark on two things. *First*, in rapidly growing children not all longitudinal bone growth occurs at the epiphyseal plates. Much of it also occurs in the depths of the cartilage covering all of their sliding joints. Where the spongy bone in the epiphyses partly protects the epiphyseal plate from unusual local concentrations of mechanical forces, the articular chondral growth regions become very much and directly exposed to such local concentrations. *Second*, at rest (and as viewed from the

Clinical Application of the Chondral Modeling Laws 149

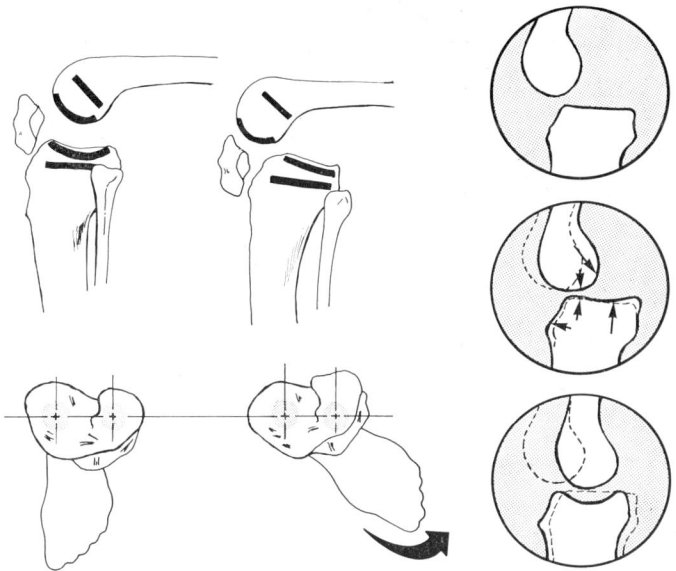

Figure 7.04. Upper left: A lateral view of the left knee to illustrate the events which the author proposes account for correction of internal tibial torsion. *Upper middle:* An external rotation splint applied to the foot moves the lateral tibial condyle rearwards (although not as much as shown here). The shaded areas (below, left and middle) on the tibial condyle show how the regions of maximum load transfer move when the splint is in use. *Right:* The ensuing changes in the pattern of chondral growth speed in the region then tend to restore good "fit" of the femoral and tibial condyles, which produces structural correction of the original malalignment of the ankle joint's plane of motion relative to that of the knee.

lateral side of the knee in this drawing) the contours of the normal tibial and femoral condyles match each other quite well (i.e. their surfaces maintain good concentricity or "fit"), so that any compression load carried by the normal joint distributes reasonably evenly over a relatively large joint surface area.

The situation of evenly distributed loading changes when Mr. Clinton or Mr. Smith of our Brace Shop applies a Fillauer or Dennis-Browne splint to turn the feet outwards, for then the anterior part of the lateral tibial condyle moves backwards to impinge on the anterior part of the lateral femoral condyle. This relieves the opened-up regions posteriorly of their normal compression loads and transfers those loads to the aforementioned impinging regions, adding to the compression loads they normally carry. This moves the chondral growth response characteristic in the impinging regions over to the descending limb of the curve in Figure 6.02. (Note: Insufficient external rotation in the splint can actually accelerate rather than retard that growth, thereby perpetuating the problem. We have observed this phenomenon in clinical practice.)

Consequently, chondral growth in the impinging regions decreases, while that in the stress-relieved regions continues normally. With further growth, and (as Dr. C. Shock has pointed out) aided by knee motion during the day and night which *over time* distributes these effects much more widely, gradually, and evenly over the joint surfaces than this static drawing implies, relocation and realignment of the joint surfaces occurs relative to the fixed bony diaphyses from which they arise and to which they remain firmly attached.

On the medial side of this knee, the opposite occurs; that is, the posterior part of the medial tibial condyle moves forward to impinge on the posterior part of the medial femoral condyle, suppressing chondral growth in that region while the stress-relieved anterior regions continue to grow.

By this rather simple means, considerable change of the rotational alignment of the growing foot relative to the growing femur can occur. Of course, changes of similar kind must occur in the ankle joint, but I believe they account for less than one-third of the total correction. Some gradual creep or plastic-like flow of the cartilaginous structures may also participate, but it tends to restore itself within a couple of months after discontinuing the splints.

Extrinsic vs. Intrinsic Forces: When a deformity stems, not from some intrinsic tissue abnormality such as a blighted local growth potential or an abnormal muscle balance arising from paralysis, spasticity, or other related cause, but rather from the action of extrinsic factors such as the fetus' position in the uterus or the infant's sleeping habits, then such a corrected deformity almost invariably remains corrected and shows no or at most a trivial tendency to recur (given also that one has removed the extrinsic factor).

However, if an intrinsic abnormality caused the deformity to begin with, it will still exist after correction of the deformity by means as just described. After removal of the splint it simply reasserts itself again, *causing the original deformity to recur.* Note that it usually does so by invoking exactly the same principles of action which allowed the original treatment to work, but by acting on the growing parts in an opposite sense to the therapeutically applied forces.

Thus the basis for a practically useful axiom in clinical orthopaedics, one stated in Volume I of this series: *Skeletal deformities of extrinsic origin rarely recur after passive correction.*

Such recurrence usually signals the existence of an intrinsic imbalance of dynamic forces acting across the endochondral growth planes of the parts. In that case, recurrences will continue to arise until one identifies and corrects the underlying intrinsic dynamic abnormality (if that is possible), or until endochondral growth ceases by virtue of increasing age or some local pathology or operative intervention. Within the last 20 years this realization has caused us to reassess and thereby to improve greatly our treatment of problems such as talipes equinovarus, spastic cerebral palsy, and congenital hip dislocation.

OTHER COMMON DEFORMITIES

Similar applications of the Chondral Modeling Laws explain the effectiveness of empirically established means of treating metatarsus adductus, club feet, genu valgum, and genu varum in infants and young children. The relations also explain the genesis of many of the skeletal deformities that occur in growing postpolio and spastic children; and in our Department of Orthopaedic Surgery specific remedial surgical procedures done on the latter early in life for such deformities (described in Volume I), procedures suggested exactly by analytical inversion of these relations, have corrected many of these problems repeatedly and consistently.

TABLE 7.02
CHONDRAL MODELING-DEPENDENT DEFORMITIES

Talipes equinovarus	Metatarsus adductus
Pes planus	Genu varum
Internal femoral torsion	Genu valgum
Internal tibial torsion	Idiopathic scoliosis
External tibial torsion	Coxa valga (true)
Spastic rocker-bottom foot	Congenital hip dysplasia
Coxa vara, congenital	Congenital dislocation of the hip
Madelung's deformity	Some limb length discrepancies (postpolio)
Internal humeral torsion (Erb's)	

This table lists a variety of children's clinical deformities and problems which the author proposes arise as the consequence of normal chondral modeling potential responding in predictable fashion to abnormal biomechanical force environments and factors, some extrinsic to the body and some intrinsic to it but still extrinsic to the affected chondral growth planes.

Table 7.02 lists some conditions of clinical importance which represent chondral modeling errors arising as consequences of the Heuter-Volkmann relations in action.

In sum, any device or procedure which concentrates appreciable compression loads on a small region of a chondral growth plane will slow down subsequent local growth predictably. So, one can use what growth potential remains plus a knowledge of the Chondral Growth Laws, plus some clinical and mechanical ingenuity to achieve better alignment of deformed parts by modifying in an appropriate manner any remaining chondral growth. Because the relative growth rate declines with age, and fairly steeply so, the younger the child the more effective and rapid this approach; the older, the less effective and slower. Clinical experience suggests that the optimum results of such treatment will occur in children under age five years, preferably under age two years. Do not forget that in idiopathic scoliosis the principle continues to function to some usable extent up to approximately age 14 years, as Dr. C. Shock and Dr. L. Z. Shifrin recently pointed out to me.

SHEARING FORCE PHENOMENA

As noted before, healthy epiphyseal plates appear relatively insensitive to compression-shearing force couples, especially if distributed relatively uniformly around their circumferences.

However, if the cartilage has abnormal mechanical quality, such shear can cause enough creep to give rise to pathological degrees of transverse displacement, as in the accompanying figure of the wrist in a child with severe renal rickets (Fig. 7.05).

Of course, sudden failure and shearing displacement can occur in response to shearing forces of traumatic origin and greatly supernormal magnitude; we term these latter problems "acute epiphysiolistheses" or "traumatic slipped epiphyses." Circumferentially nonuniform shear of physiologic amount (that is, an unusual shearing resultant in a given direction as occurs normally in the knee and hip) can cause very slow sideways displacement of a normal epiphysis, but this occurs so slowly relative to the speed of longitudinal growth and subsequent bony replacement of the newly produced cartilage that it rarely leads to pathological deformities. The low coefficient of friction of the normal joint-lubricating mechanisms (the drag of which provides the major source of the shearing forces acting on epiphyseal plates) and normal anatomical configurations and relationships probably quite effectively protect planes of endochondral growth from harmful amounts of shear. The shear-related problems we do encounter in clinical practice seem to involve hyaline cartilage of grossly abnormal mechanical properties (slipped capital femoral epiphyses, the chondrodystrophies, various forms of primary and secondary rickets). (See Aegerter and Kirkpatrick,[1] Rubin.[79])

MODELING AND REMODELING

Joint Architecture and Cartilage Modeling

This term signifies structurally functional adaptations, initiated and controlled partly by factors inherent in the tissue and partly by the biomechanical milieu of the tissue. We just finished describing some effects of the growth/force-response characteristic that endow growing chondral tissue with the modeling (i.e. archi-

154 *The Physiology of Cartilaginous, Fibrous, and Bony Tissue*

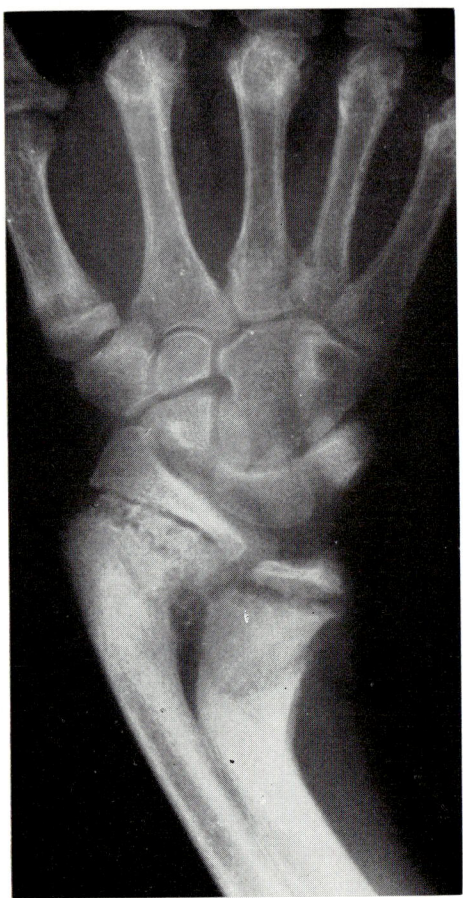

Figure 7.05. This teen-aged child had severe and protracted renal failure leading to secondary hyperparathyroidism and so-called "renal rickets." He developed widespread bony deformities representing shearing displacements of various epiphyseal plates; one view of one wrist shown here demonstrates ulnarwards displacement of both radial and ulnar epiphyses. This represents the effects of normal shearing forces acting on an epiphyseal plate of abnormal mechanical properties.

tectural adaptive) capability. In that respect one thing more remains to be said, which I will introduce in the form of a question.

Why is the knee a hinge joint and the hip a ball and socket? For decades, the standard answer held that these properties represent fairly direct effects of genetic predetermination inherent in the local cartilage cells and their progenitor cells at the time of conception. (See Enlow[24] for a thoughtful discussion of this problem.) I now suggest a major modification of that view, as follows:

I propose that the hip becomes a ball-and-socket joint simply because the *anatomy and function of its musculature* subject it to ball-and-socket motions from its inception; given that embryologically determined fact (of course, one ultimately determined by genetic factors but now those more remote ones that determine muscle alignment, attachment, and contractural patterns), the Chondral Modeling Laws subsequently *had* to create a ball-and-socket configuration of the hip joint.

I propose that the knee becomes a hinge joint simply because from its inception in the embryo its musculature functions in such a way as to subject it only to hinge-like motions; accordingly, it developed contours at its growing and opposing chondral surfaces which permitted such motion. A preceding figure illustrated beautifully what can happen to a hinge joint (the ankle) if, quite early in life, it becomes subjected to unusually large ball-and-socket type mechanical forces.

I propose that the radiohumeral joint has exactly those contours which allow hinge motion plus rotation of the radius around its longitudinal axis, simply because it was endowed with motors (and neurologic coordinating patterns) which forced exactly such motions on these parts during their development in the embryo, fetus, and infant; by the Chondral Modeling Laws the structure adapted to fill that need, i.e. the growing chondral planes produced exactly those shapes which would allow the muscles free play.

Cartilage Turnover

Cartilage does undergo a kind of turnover throughout its existence, although of a primarily chemical nature, where in the case of bone it represents actual cellular and tissue turnover occasioned by different kinds of cooperating cells which actively and first solubilize a small amount or "packet" ($\approx .05\text{mm}^3$) of bony tissue and then replace it with newly made stuff.

In the case of healthy cartilage, turnover of the MPS (chondroitin sulfates A and C) occurs relatively rapidly, according to Henry Mankin[59] requiring about eight days in a rabbit and probably on the order of three months in an adult man. The turnover process accelerates greatly in response to local injuries such as a fracture entering the joint, a cut in its surface made by a surgeon, or the pounding taken by a local joint area when the joint surface has become rough and irregular as the result of degenerative joint disease, trauma, or the residue of rheumatoid arthritis. Such injuries usually also lead to a great increase in the local chondroblast division rate.

While some students of such matters have denied it categorically, I nevertheless agree with Moffett *et al*[69] that in uninjured adult cartilage a slow rate of annual turnover probably occurs of both the MPS and the collagen, and that a slow, basal rate of chondroblast division occurs too, so that in a year's time approximately one per cent of the collagen and cells become replaced. I visualize this turnover as providing a *maintenance mechanism* which repairs damage associated with the normal daily wear and tear of actively used joints. In other words, I propose that the practical operational immunity exhibited to mechanical fatigue by joint cartilage arises not by producing mechanically perfect structural materials (elementary observations demonstrate that they are *not* perfect in this sense) but rather by equipping them with cellularly based active mechanisms that could (a) *detect* such damage while it still remains microscopic (and thus trivial) in extent, (b) then *remove* that damaged material, (c) and finally *replace* it with new undamaged material intimately bonded to the preexisting structures.

Parenthetically, those who seek, for use in the human body, a strong adhesive which can retain its strength in an aequeous ionic environment really ran far afield when they applied for and obtained federal funds to study how barnacles attach to rocks and ship hulls. The so-called cementing or reversal lines present in the bones of all species of mammalian, avian, and teleost skeletons *represent exactly such an adhesive,* one already perfectly tailored in the chemical, immunologic, and biological senses to our own internal milieu, and demonstrably as durable as the bone itself. To use a more obviously silly analogy, if one wants to study the role of chlorophyll in photosynthesis, why try to go to the planet Venus to do it?

Cartilage Creep

To repeat, when subjected to shearing forces over considerable periods of time, both hyaline and fibrocartilage undergo a slow kind of yielding or flowing which mechanical engineers call "creep." Since the collagen fibers flow to a lesser degree than the MPS-water gel embedding them, these fibrils tend to stretch out and align themselves parallel to the direction of creep. One can observe a good analogy in the alignment of seaweed in an incoming tide. I discuss some of the biomechanical properties of this phenomenon elsewhere and will only mention two of them here.

In essence, this creep allows collagen fibers in the cartilaginous surfaces of joints to align parallel to the direction of greatest relative motion of the two joint surfaces; that automatically provides those surfaces great strength to disruption in shear and tangential tension.

Creep also provides a purely passive and nonbiologic means for relieving a small joint region or incongruity that carries too much load locally.

SOME OBSERVATIONAL BACKGROUND FOR THIS MODEL

In effect, the preceding material presented a theory of how biomechanical factors influence both the overall direction and the local speed of chondral growth. Others have attempted to construct analogous models in the past, and in many details such models predict rather different things than the one you just read. It may interest the curious reader to know the observational basis for the various points in this model and for its relatively laconic and nondefensive statement. I know the following from some previous personal experience with model building as a general problem: (a) This model is at least essentially correct but, (b) it puts things so differently from others' previous ones and from the constructs found in contemporary literature that many will find it hard to grasp in the first reading (for example, see Smith[87]), while (c) others will ridicule it, deny it, or even totally ignore it (the ultimate "worse" for any author or model-builder).

Two observations apply here. First, some people still believe the earth is flat, a truly remarkable testimonial (in this day of pictures taken from satellites and by astronauts) to the ability of the brain to insulate itself from the meanings of facts.

Second, we remember who burned Rome, not who built it. From the viewpoint of participants in this action, however, the building act provides more (and more immediate) satisfaction than Nero probably finds in the fact that nearly 1500 years later you and I know who he was.

The basis of this model represents (a) common-sense analysis and (b) billions of beautifully and exquisitely controlled experiments run repeatedly in different areas, nations, cultures, and climates and observed repeatedly by many thousands of inquisitive minds athirst to understand and verily burning to justify in terms of augmented medical understanding the enormous private and federal expense of conducting those experiments.

I refer, of course, to the perfectly normal growing child or other mammal, and specifically to his skeletal patterns of growth. To illustrate some of its features important to the argument, I will refer to common clinical knowledge as well as to the x-rays of the pelvis and the hips of a skeletally healthy child shown in Figure 7.06. The following paragraphs will deal separately with the effects of compression and tension loading on chondral growth.

Compression

Clinicians know that when a chondral growth plane carries too much compression load, chondral growth stops. We sometimes achieve this deliberately by bracketing a chondral growth plane with a set of Dr. W. Blount's staples or by inserting a bone graft across an epiphyseal plate which, when it heals to the spongy bone

Clinical Application of the Chondral Modeling Laws

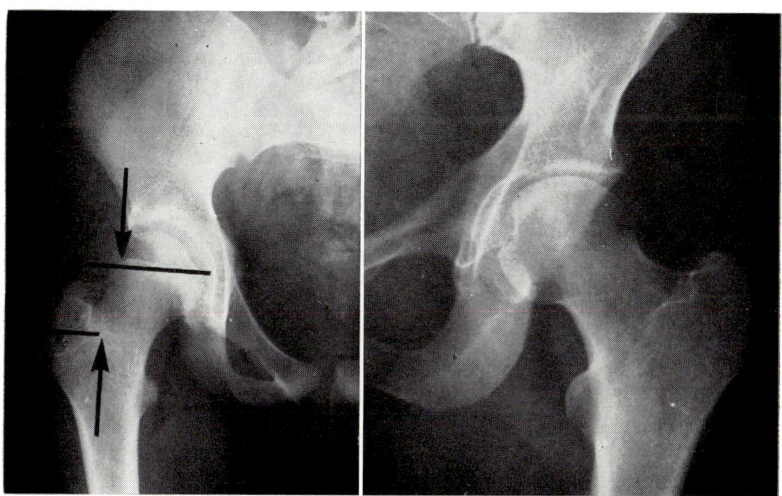

Figure 7.06. AP x-ray of the hips of a skeletally normal child on the left. The horizontal black lines define the vertical distance between the capital femoral epiphyseal plate, which carries a compression load throughout growth, and the greater trochanteric epiphyseal plate, which carries a tension load. The vertical distance between them (identified by the arrows) increases by approximately 2 cm from early childhood to skeletal maturity around age 18 years, as shown in the x-ray of an adult hip on the right. The author submits that this situation (a sizeable number of other and comparable ones exist in the body; all show this same behavior) should resolve the argument as to whether cartilage grows faster in compression than in tension, or conversely.

on the epiphyseal and metaphyseal sides of the plate, then acts as a kind of biological staple. Furthermore, we know that given too few staples or too small a bone graft, the pressure from the growth plate can break these structures or extrude the staples, allowing growth to resume. It requires no great erudition (or risk of error) to extrapolate from those facts to this idea: As one increases the compression load from the normal physiological range towards that level which leads to total arrest of chondral growth, one should obtain a range of gradually increasing degrees of retardation before total arrest occurs. Hence, the basic shape of the right-hand side or *descending limb* of the curve in Figure 6.02.

Now regard another revealing situation. Of the billions of adults alive in the world today, surprisingly few developed pathological degrees of genu valgum or genu varum.

With respect to Sherlock Holmes' "dog that did not bark"—that is, the many thousands of persons who did not develop malalignments of their knees during growth for each one who did (without some recognized underlying metabolic bone disease)—the insight of cybernetics can help. When any given dynamic parameter almost never varies beyond trivial limits in a dynamic system that provides plenty of opportunity for it to do so (here, in the presence of major changes in size and growth speed), the experienced control system engineer infers that *something within the system actively controls that parameter*, in such a way as to minimize, and actively and aggressively correct any error. In such situations a control system almost invariably proves to exist and constitutes a negative feedback system, in that any "error" in the controlled parameter itself stimulates the activity leading to its correction. Corrective activity stops when correction has been attained because that very attainment then eliminates the corrective stimulus.

That point of view plus previously recorded facts imply a negative feedback relationship affecting chondral growth speed across epiphyseal plates. Hence, I place the physiologic midpoint of the chondral growth-response characteristic or curve slightly onto the left of its peak, and on the *ascending limb* of the curve in Figure 6.02 rather than at its peak. Confirmation of the accuracy of this choice comes from two other sources: our experience with postpolio children and the relationship between the growth rates of tension and compression loaded chondral growth regions (i.e. epiphyses and apophyses) in the same bone.

With respect to the former, when a limb was paralyzed so that muscle forces were removed but orthotic support allowed the child to bear weight, we commonly observed retardation in longitudinal growth of the affected compared to the normal side. Of course, this fact alone does not *prove* that losing the extra compression loads of the muscles on the paralyzed side was responsible for that either directly or ultimately, because one could argue alternatively that changes in blood flow associated with the postpolio effects on the sympathetic nervous system might cause this retardation. Partly or wholly I would counter that with the observation that length discrepancies have not proven an important and predictable postsympathectomy problem, whether done in human children for other purposes or in experimental animals to prove (or disprove) the present point. We do not really need this particular argument, for another and self-sufficient one exists and comes up in the next paragarph. While the same point relative to growth retardation could be made for similar circumstances found in myelodysplasia and some other forms of cerebral palsy, one could also raise the same objections to them, so I would propose such situations as circumstantial supporting evidence rather than proof of my point. The most convincing evidence to my mind (the reader certainly is not obligated to agree) includes the "dog that did not bark," already mentioned, and the situation discussed next.

Tension

Some theorists have proposed that (as compared to compression) tension accelerates chondral growth, and one certainly could see the intuitive logic of that proposition. However, relative to the hip x-ray in Figure 7.06 note the following indisputable facts:

1. The capital femoral epiphyseal plate carries a compression load throughout its existence.

2. The epiphyseal plate of the greater trochanter carries a tension load throughout its period of existence.

3. In the infant, the epiphyseal plate of the head lies only a couple of centimeters higher than that of the greater trochanter.

4. By age 15 or so when these plates have closed, the capital femoral epiphyseal plate (or its residue) lies some four to five centimeters higher than the epiphyseal plate of the greater trochanter.

5. Obviously, then, over the intervening years the capital plate grew faster than the plate of the greater trochanter; i.e. *the compression-loaded plate grew faster than the tension-loaded plate.*

> QED: Chondral planes grow faster under physiologic compression loading than under physiologic tension loading.

The observation that while the greater trochanter grows nearly vertically, the capital epiphysis grows medially as well as vertically further reenforces that conclusion, for in terms of total centimeters of growth, the latter must grow an extra bit more than any increase it adds to vertical height alone.

Numerous examples exist in growing skeletons of other compression-tension—loaded pairs of chondral growth planes, and as far as I can see they all support the conclusion just drawn. Hence the shape and slope of the ascending limb or left-hand part of the curve in Figure 6.02.

Comment: Why have experimentalists not succeeded in demonstrating such effects in laboratory animals? The pertinent reasons seem simple and few.

First, the growing child provides the final and authoritative experiment, done repeatedly and under completely natural conditions, but few scientists in our basic science field have learned to accept that fact and, even more important, how to make productive use of it. Obviously, in such a situation one should use animal experimentation to try to understand *how* these things happen but not to demonstrate the basic nature of *what.*

Second, in most such experiments surgical procedures were performed and/or artificial devices inserted in bones or in or across joints. These introduce considerable soft and bony tissue injury, which consistently and predictably leads to an acceleration of remodeling, subsequent growth, and adaptation in all of the tissues in the region, as I described a few years ago.[34] In bone, I called it a *posttraumatic osteodystrophy;* here, the important fact lies in that a quite analogous phenomenon affects all of the regional tissue structures, including the cartilage and fibrous tissue structures. It normally requires several *months* for that injury-triggered activity to subside; until it does, any experimental observations almost surely will relate to the surgical trauma rather than to additional factors such as stress, piezoelectrical currents, or drugs.

In other words, an operation itself introduces an additional variable into the system, one of sufficient magnitude as to challenge in a major way all of the local tissue systems, and to which (in the absence of certain diseases*) they all respond rather dramatically and consistently. That many experimentalists have worked in ignorance of this or even have chosen to disbelieve it has not by one iota diminished its disturbing effects on their experiments and thus on their interpretations of results.

WHY AND HOW?

By what means does compression and/or tension affect chondral growth speed? Does it do so by altering the cell division frequencies in the germinal layer? By altering the amount of new cartilage matrix synthesized per chondroblast? Whichever the case, does it do so by some direct effect on these activities, by altering their nutrition, or by altering their sensitivity to circulating regulatory factors, such as hormones and/or vitamins?

How do these forces affect chondral growth direction (apart from examples given in the preceding chapter in which regional variations in growth speed cause predictable tilting of chondral growth planes)? By inducing creep of the material, by altering cellular behavior, or both?

These seem to provide cogent questions for research into spatial polarization of cartilage growth in the coming years.

QUESTIONS

1. In terms of the Chondral Modeling Laws, explain the genesis of vertebral wedging in a severe case of idiopathic scoliosis.
2. In the same terms, explain the development of shortening of the growing lower limbs (a) in myelomeningocele, (b) after paralysis by poliomyelitis, (c) after sciatic nerve palsy due to nerve transection in childhood, (d) in spastic cerebral palsy.

---

*These diseases include advanced diabetes mellitus—especially when some neuropathy also exists—and tertiary lues.

164 *The Physiology of Cartilaginous, Fibrous, and Bony Tissue*

3. Reduction of congenital hip dislocation before age 18 months usually leads to a good hip; after age 36 months it rarely does. Why?
4. Adults who underwent hip arthrodesis in childhood usually have lax knee ligaments on the ipsilateral side; those who undergo it in adult life usually do not or develop much less of it. Why?
5. About two-thirds of the club feet we see correct readily and display little tendency to recur, thereby making us look good. One-third, however, do not correct readily and tend to recur as long as growth continues. What do these differences tell you about their causes? About the means of treatment needed to master them? What you may reasonably expect of your therapeutic efforts?

Chapter VIII

Biomechanical Response Characteristics of Fibrous Tissue

Like bone, fibrous tissue arises, functions, and usually endures well enough that men die of malfunctions arising in other tissues. Its physiology poses the problems of understanding its creation, growth, physical and structural properties, adaptations to mechanical and chemical factors, its repair, changes related to aging, the nature of its internal maintenance activity, its role in the body's economy, and finally its diseases. This chapter considers chiefly its biodynamic responses to mechanical forces and selected properties of its repair and turnover activities.

The subjects of little attention in our existing literature and perhaps one of my real contributions to orthopaedic basic sciences, the biodynamic force-response properties and characteristics of skeletal tissues, nevertheless directly concern and interest all clinical orthopaedists.

Observe in terms of our skeletal alphabet that, in adding the behavioral letter "fibrous tissue production" to the new functional letters representing its biomechanical responses to mechanical tension loads, we can create several entirely new functional words. Let us first define some of those functions and then describe how they are realized.

Before doing so, note that Figure 8.01 relates the content of this chapter to overall skeletal physiology.

FIBROUS TISSUE FUNCTIONS

Living tendon, ligament, and fascia exhibit several very simple but highly useful responses to biomechanical factors, which as-

TABLE 8.01
ABBREVIATIONS USED IN CHAPTER VIII

STH: Somatotrophic hormone; growth hormone

166 *The Physiology of Cartilaginous, Fibrous, and Bony Tissue*

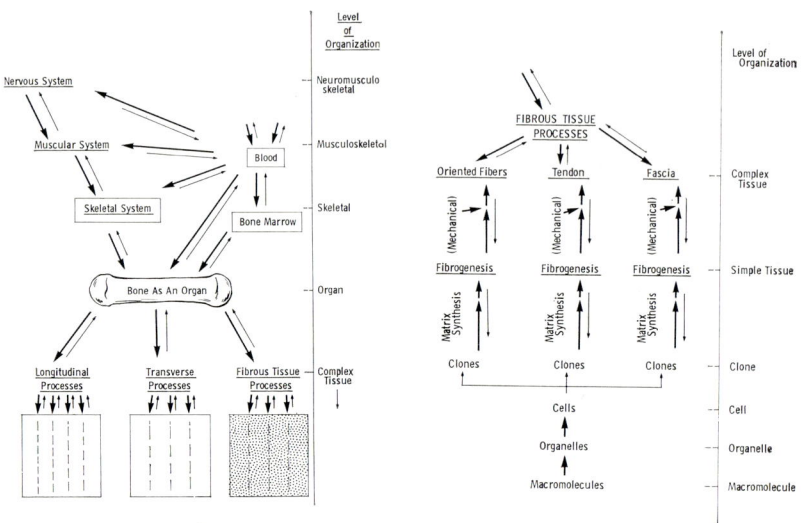

Figure 8.01. The hatched area locates the subject matter of this chapter within the overall scheme of neuromusculoskeletal physiology.

sume relevance and meaning only when placed in the focus of the basic functions such structures and tissues exist to provide. The functions are as follows:

1. The collagen fibers present in and characteristic of all fibrous tissues exist to provide great rigidity and strength to tension or stretching loads aligned parallel to the long axis of the fibers (their first-order function). In engineering jargon they exist to provide a high tension modulus of elasticity or low compliance in tension.

2. Fibrous tissue in bulk possesses some mechanism which brings most of its individual fiber bundles into alignment parallel with the tension loads it carries, thereby promoting maximum tensile strength with a minimum amount of collagen.

3. Fibrous tissues possessing such spatial order and alignment, while providing great tensile strength in that direction, permit flexibility (i.e. high compliance) in all other orientations, which includes both shear and compression relative to the longitudinal axes of their component fibers and fibrils (another first-order function).

4. These mechanical properties permit the construction of

thread-like and rope-like structures (tendons, ligaments) intended to carry unidirectional mechanical tension loads.

5. These properties also permit the construction of two-dimensional fabric-like structures, some of which carry directly applied and parallel-aligned tension loads (iliotibial tract, interosseous membranes, the lacertus fibrosus), others of which contain perpendicularly aligned bursting-type loads (fascia enveloping large arteries and veins, and organs such as the kidney, liver, and muscle), and yet others which bind elements of other tissue types into purposeful anatomical structures (fascial investment of peripheral nerves).

6. Living structures made of bulk fibrous tissue possess a separate mechanism that adapts and matches their size (and thus their strength) to the tension loads they characteristically carry.

Fibrous tissue acts like a phylogenetically more primitive and elementary substance and structural material than either kinds of cartilage or bone. If we see only a dim but essentially correct outline of our own evolution, fibrous tissue must have evolved long before hard tissues. This primitiveness seems to appear in a variety of ways in clinical practice. For example, one type of fracture nonunion often seen these days represents a kind of biological failure in that the tissues in the region of the fracture seemingly cannot produce functionally competent osteoblasts or chondroblasts, and so the fracture does not heal. But scar (i.e. fibrous tissue) still does arise in at least some quantities in such a fracture.

Functionally speaking, the individual fibers of fibrous tissue indeed resemble man-made thread, for from threads we make string and from string we make rope (analogous to tendon or ligament) to obtain tensile rigidity and strength along only one direction or axis; we also weave fabrics (analogous to fascia) out of threads which supply tensile rigidity in two directions lying in a common plane, while retaining essentially complete flexibility in all orientations under shearing and compression loads. I will term the biodynamic properties that allow fibrous tissue to fulfill such functions as the "stretch-hypertrophy law," the "curvature rule," and the "stretch-creep law," all as far as I know my own brain children.

168 *The Physiology of Cartilaginous, Fibrous, and Bony Tissue*

The following paragraphs will deal with these operational rules and will not deal with the mechanism that causes the collagen fibrils in fibrous tissue to align parallel to the local tension resultant (because I do not know its identity).

BIOMECHANICAL RESPONSE CHARACTERISTICS

The Stretch Hypertrophy Law

Living collagenous tissue structures react to excessive *intermittent tension* parallel to the collagen fibers comprising their major bulk by increasing their cross-section area in a plane perpendicular to the direction of tension, as shown in the accompanying Figure 8.02. This build-up in diameter or, more accurately, in cross-section area occurs when the fibrocytes residing in the tissue undergo activation following abnormally large elongations due to abnormally large tension loads (for example, as in growing children, with growing muscles and thus progressively increasing tension loads) and then produce the new collagen whose fibers align parallel to the tension load resultant acting on the part during their deposition. Note by way of emphasis that increasing the cross-section area of a tendon (or ligament) perpendicularly to its anatomical length should increase its tensile strength (and total tensile rigidity) nearly in direct proportion. Normally, the increase in cross-section area would continue until the total strength of the organ reduced its actual physical elongation or stretch under those tension loads below some physiologic minimum level, which probably lies somewhere below approximately 2 per cent of the structure's maximum length (technically, such stretch in tension constitutes tension *strain*). Once it attains the required strength further hypertrophy ceases simply because that strength itself eliminates the generation of tension-induced activating and differentiating signals to the tendon cells. If given time, fibrous tissues apparently can increase in cross-section area in this fashion nearly without limit to meet such situations.

We may phrase this principle of action, which I call the "Stretch Hypertrophy Law," in the following words:

Intermittent stretch causes collagenous tissues to hypertrophy,

Biomechanical Response Characteristics of Fibrous Tissue

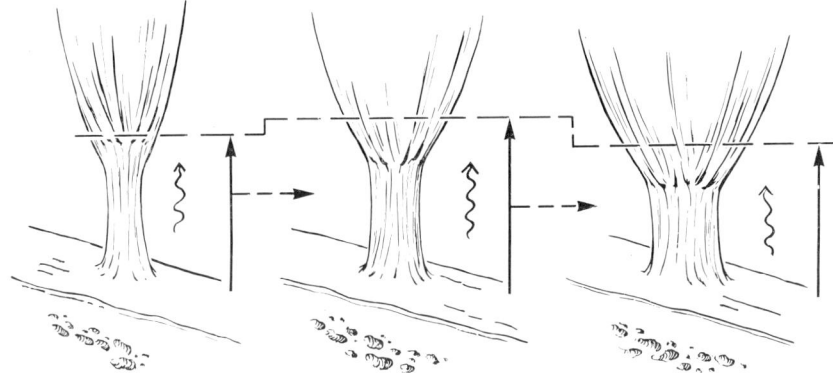

Figure 8.02. The Stretch-Hypertrophy Law in action. *Left:* A tendon transmitting the tension load of a contracting muscle (above) to a bone (below). The vertical large arrows each represents tendon length during a contraction of the muscle, and the wavy arrows indicate the tendon length that accompanies each relaxation, i.e. its resting length. *Middle:* The muscle increases in strength (and bulk too) as a result of STH effect during growth and/or exercise. Note that the amount of stretch with each contraction has now increased. I propose that this provides the basic stimulus that activates and makes the tendon cell system begin to produce more collagen that ultimately does the following: *Right:* It increases the diameter and cross-section area of the tendon, and thus its total strength, until once more the total amount of stretch with each contraction reduces to its original (and physiologic) amount.

until the resulting increase in strength reduces elongation in tension to some minimum level.

In an earlier monograph, I term this the "minimum effective strain,"[33] meaning that amount of deformation insufficient to set the adapting system in motion. That concept looks better and better with the passage of years, particularly the essentially stochastic base I built it on.

Qualifications

1. In some manner this adaptive property of fibrous tissue *averages tension loads over some period of time.* The hypertrophic

response to excessive stretch probably represents a reaction more to that overall average than it does to occasional but unusually large forces. The duration of the averaging period remains unknown (I do not believe it has yet occurred to anyone to try to measure it) but probably approximates three to nine months, based on circumstantial clinical evidence. One clinical clue to this period arises with successful ligament or tendon grafting; one should spend at least three to nine months (and probably some multiple of this) in gradually increasing loading before expecting it to sustain full loads.

2. *A series of repeated tension loads, not a single one and not a constant one, cause this rule to become operative.* Single loads probably cause no significant biological changes, while constant loads receive further attention shortly.

3. *Decreasing the typical stretching loads on these tissues does not cause their cross-section area to decrease.* In other words, the build-up referred to acts like a one-way street. However, if severe and protracted, such load reduction can lead to some edema of the structure and to impaired lateral cohesiveness of its individual collagen fibers; these changes could greatly weaken the overall structure.

4. *The capacity to hypertrophy in response to excessive stretch depends upon the presence within the fibrous tissue structure in question of viable fibrocytes and of a patent blood supply.* I believe this explains, at least in part, why attempts to make new ligaments out of free fascial or tendon grafts often fail: Function, meaning carrying tension loads, often resumes so soon after the operation that the bulk of the still-dead graft has insufficient cells to respond and to cause diametric hypertrophy fast enough to maintain itself without elongating in fatigue. Drs. E. Guise and D. C. Mitchell have used this idea in modifying their treatment of athletic injuries to major ligaments, with some considerable success.

Table 8.02 summarizes the major features of fibrous tissue physiology which underly its force-response characteristics.

TABLE 8.02
THE BASIS OF FIBROUS TISSUE (IN THE COMPLEX SENSE) PHYSIOLOGY FROM THE BIOMECHANICAL STANDPOINT

Morphological events	Appearance of fibroblasts; appearance of collagen with fibers aligned with tension loads.
Behavioral events and processes	Mesenchymal cell activation → proliferation → differentiation of fibroblasts → secretion of hyaluronic acid plus collagen → turnover.
Functions	To carry tension loads—as threads, ropes, fabric, and volume-containing investments; to resist mechanical fatigue failure; to increase in bulk according to size of tension loads; growth.

In terms of the alphabet concept this table summarizes the basic structural, behavioral, and functional properties of complex fibrous tissues as they appear in normal tendon, ligament, and fascia.

The following word diagram epitomizes the essential interactions envisioned in this system:

STRETCH-HYPERTROPHY LAW:

(Fibrogenetic cells) ⇌ *(Collagen Fibers)* ⇌ *(Mechanical Stretch)*

Comment: This law would explain the clinical observation that the tensile strength of each tendon normally matches exactly the time-averaged contractile force (not the same thing in physics as power) of the muscle that actuates it. Were this law not true, then it should follow that spontaneous tendon ruptures associated with mismatched tendon strength-muscle force situations should form a common clinical entity. Although such failures do occur they remain very uncommon, for each represents well over 100,000,000 tendon load-deload cycles per failure in the population at large. Thus, again, a "dog that did not bark."

I propose, in part to explain that missing bark, that as a muscle's contractile force increases during growth, the progressively increasing tension loads and strains it applies to its tendon stimulate an increase in the latter's cross-section area according to the Stretch-Hypertrophy Law. When muscle growth ceases, then shortly thereafter the diametric growth of tendon should do so also (it does).

Then, in effect, I argue that *function determines structure*. If true, it should follow that a muscle weakened early in childhood by paralytic disease, such as poliomyelitis or muscular dystrophy, should attach to a tendon proportionally reduced in cross-section area (this is true). Note that were the diametric growth of a tendon directly determined, not by the stretch hypertrophy rule but instead by systemic factors such as STH acting directly on the tendon fibroblasts or by genetic factors inherent in the tenoblasts themselves, growth should continue even after the muscle became paralyzed. Observation reveals that it does not.

This principle of action also should cause each joint ligament to increase in cross-section area until it provides the amount of tensile strength needed to stabilize joints during active function. Likewise, it should cause fascial sheaths to hypertrophy as required to withstand the tensile and/or expansile forces acting upon them, of which the condensation in the deep fascia of the lateral thigh known as the iliotibial tract affords an excellent example.

Finally, this law explains the hypertrophying contractures of the dermis of the skin, which follow longitudinal incisions made across the flexor aspects of joints.

The Curvature Rule

The deceptively simple Stretch-Hypertrophy Law exhibits one peculiar but important behavioral characteristic that governs its response in the presence of a curvature in its anatomical trajectory or path. (A related effect described in Volume IV of this series appears in bone modeling behavior.) This characteristic appears most clearly in skin incisions. Specifically, and like any other fibrous tissue, a longitudinal scar will hypertrophy in response to intermittent tension, *if and only if* (a) that tension occurs in a straight-line pull, or (b) if running across a curved surface, its trajectory presents its *concave* side towards the external surface of the skin. Otherwise, the following *curvature rule* applies:

The ability to hypertrophy exhibits inhibition when a curving scar presents its convex side towards the skin.

Thus, given a longitudinal incision crossing the concave, flexor aspect of the elbow joint (or finger or knee or whatever), extending such joints momentarily stretches the scar, its dermal side has a concave curvature, and (as the above rule predicts) that intermittent stretch will stimulate additional collagen production by fibroblasts, i.e. the original incisional scar will hypertrophy.

A longitudinal scar crossing the convex *extensor* aspect of the elbow (or knee or finger or any other joint) presents its convex side towards the skin which, according to this rule, will inhibit hypertrophy of the scar. Clinical observation repeatedly demonstrates these effects.

I do not understand what biological and/or physical-chemical factors cause the stretch-hypertrophy behavior, although clearly some means must exist to activate and "instruct" the local fibroblasts and their progenitor cells in these situations. These form important problems for future research. While we have many questions and few answers at this writing, this ignorance should not cloud the fact that the operational behavior described above is highly reproducible and dependable in clinical practice, i.e. one can depend that the Stretch-Hypertrophy Law will predict correctly.

The Stretch-Creep Rule

When loaded in *constant tension*, living collagenous tissues exhibit mechanical creep. The term "creep" applies to the mechanical properties of structural materials and signifies a very gradual, progressive, and nonelastic yielding of the material to some mechanical load imposed on it from without. In spite of such creep, the material may remain quite strong and relatively unyielding to suddenly applied loads of brief duration, even when very large.

The opening sentence means that under the influence of continuous gentle tension loads, living collagenous structures gradually stretch out or elongate. This phenomenon may explain why a wedging cast or other forms of gentle but constant traction can correct flexion contractures of knees, elbows, hips, fingers, and ankles, even when attempts to do so quickly and by brute force would either rupture the fibrous bands or, more likely, break the underlying bones.

Figure 8.03 (top) shows a dramatic example of this creep at work in response to continuous traction.

174 *The Physiology of Cartilaginous, Fibrous, and Bony Tissue*

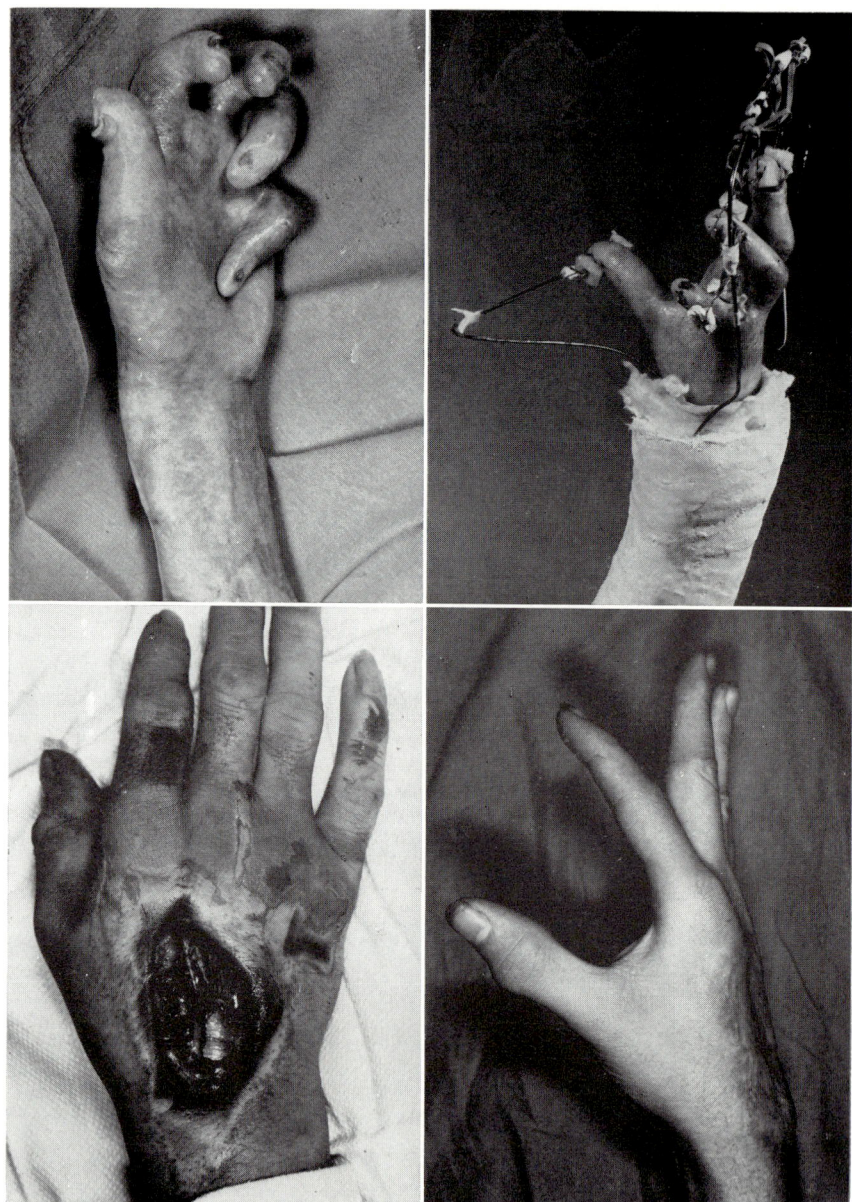

Figure 8.03. Top left: A badly burned hand, months after coverage by multiple split-thickness grafts. Severe and rigid flexion contractures and arthrofibrosis affect all MP and IP joints. *Top right:* After 14 days in gentle

The preceding statements seem to me to imply that some creep should also occur during normal function, i.e. during the intermittent tension loading which such structures carry during life. If so, then the fact that normally and in the gross anatomical sense structures such as tendons and ligaments do not elongate progressively with aging implies in its turn a *creep compensatory mechanism* which tends continuously to make up for the creep by shortening the structure. Furthermore, the fact that overshortening occurs no more than undershortening again implies some type of negative feedback mode use and flow of "information" between the creep process and the shortening mechanism, feedback such that too much creep somehow stimulates extra take-up of the elongational slack produced thereby. Such a contractural mechanism might have caused the fascial and capsular contractures which we used to see in polio children, particularly in the days when constant splinting rather than daily passive ranges of motion formed the accepted mode of therapy. One can still see such contractures in limbs continuously casted for many months. Perhaps, too, the gradual and inherent contraction of fresh wound scars and scars arising from healing by secondary intention reflect the action of such a take-up activity.

One might deliberately invoke the Stretch-Hypertrophy Law in order to generate collagenous tissue which could serve as tendon graft material for certain reconstructive problems, particular-

---

rubber-band skeletal traction. While the contractures were strong enough to have caused bony fractures had an attempt been made to extend them by manual manipulation, the constant traction caused them to creep progressively and dramatically. *Bottom left:* A third-degree burn which completely eliminated the extensor tendons to digits 2, 3, and 4. The surgeon on this case took his cue from the author and allowed it to granulate to generate some scar; he then covered it with split-thickness graft and, following healing of the graft, started the patient on repeated active range-of-motion exercises. *Bottom right:* Nine months later he had formed functionally satisfactory tendons out of that scar, and only some lag in the index required a reefing procedure for its extensor tendon. Note: these rules work clinically and in the operational sense. (Cases courtesy of John Ditmars, M. D., Division of Plastic Surgery, Henry Ford Hospital.)

ly in the hand. For example, one might deliberately make a longitudinal incision across the flexor aspect of a normal elbow, knee, or axilla, subject it to intermittent daily passive stretch, and three or more months later (and possibly repeatedly if the need existed) "harvest" the resulting subcutaneous "tendon" for use as an autogenous tendon graft. Once the reconstructive program was completed, a conventional Z plasty of the donor site should then correct the contractural problem. Such a procedure would have at least one useful property: It would eliminate any possibility of immunologic rejection one might fear in doing homografts and heterografts. Note, incidentally, that Z plasty cures the problem of incisional contractures by orienting the concavity in the angle of the "Z" so that it lies parallel to, rather than perpendicular to, the plane of the skin surface, i.e. it converts it instead to a process of horizontal folding and unfolding.

Table 8.03 summarizes the biomechanical response characteristics of fibrous tissue.

TABLE 8.03

BIOMECHANICAL RESPONSE CHARACTERISTICS OF FIBROUS TISSUE

1. Intermittent stretch causes cross-sectional growth of fibrous tissue organs until their increased strength reduces elongation below some physiologic minimum level.
2. Constant stretch causes elongational creep of fibrous tissue.
3. When stretched across curved paths, the Stretch-Hypertrophy Rule becomes inactivated on the convex side.

FIBROUS TISSUE REPAIR AND REMODELING

As holds true for bone, the fundamental differences in the processes of repairing injury to fibrous tissues on the one hand, and on the other of elaborating and maintaining them in a mechanically competent state throughout adult life have not yet received their due in our teaching literature. The following paragraphs outline some of the major features and differences of these processes.

Fibrous Tissue Repair

This repair occurs in two major stages, the initial repair and the remodeling stages.

Initial Repair

When fibrous tissue structures become grossly cut, torn, or badly contused, their vascular and perivascular cells (whether in a tendon, ligament, fascia, or the dermis) begin to proliferate to produce new capillaries and then new fibroblasts. The former invade any clot and serum occupying any soft tissue defect; the latter, when they appear, begin to synthesize new collagen and hyaluronic acid, both of which assemble and combine externally to the cell membrane of the fibroblast that made them. This collagen synthesis accompanies the elaboration of an alkaline phosphatase enzyme by the fibroblast. Parenthetically, this enzyme associates so consistently with the extracellular polymerization of collagen and in bone and cartilage as well as in soft tissues that I propose it may actually play some important role in that polymerization.

To return to repair in the structural sense, the fibers of the freshly produced mature mass of scar (called "tendon callus" if it occurs in a tendon but exactly the same in its structural and chemical details when it occurs in dermis, ligament, and fascia) lack uniform orientation, so that under a stereomicroscope they form an anarchic or spatially disorganized feltwork, the fibers running in all directions. This situation resembles that which exists at the conclusion of the initial stage in fracture repair, in which, from the mechanical load-bearing viewpoint, a spatially disorganized mass of trabeculae of mineralized fibrous bone, termed "fracture callus," has been produced. Alike for the cases of both fibrous tissue and fracture repair, at this stage musculoskeletal function can resume. Subsequent events in the healing process then continue for months or even years after all local symptoms and dysfunction have resolved and in the presence of (and possibly caused and guided by) apparently normal mechanical function and demands.

178 The Physiology of Cartilaginous, Fibrous, and Bony Tissue

Remodeling of the Callus

After function can resume, a reorganization or replacement of the fresh scar commences which in effect removes most of the original anarchic collagenous feltwork and replaces it with more newly deposited collagen fibers, *which become aligned parallel to the tension loads carried by the part.* The physicochemical mechanisms responsible for such alignment remain unknown but form an important problem for future research (if interested in first approximation ideas, see Bassett[10]). This parallel alignment provides much greater total tension strength per unit mass of collagen than does the feltwork alignment, for in the former practically all of the collagen fibers share the tension loads; in the latter those fibers lying perpendicularly to the load carry none of it, those halfway between perpendicular and parallel carry only a fraction of it, while only those relatively few fibers accurately parallel to the load carry the brunt of it. (see Fig. 8.04.) Since

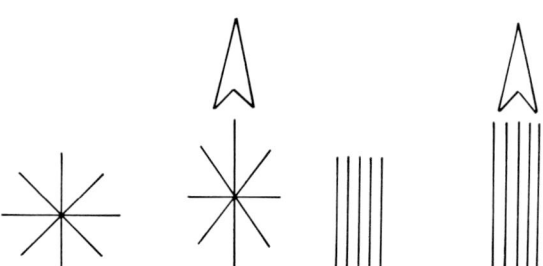

Figure 8.04. Left: An anarchic mass of fibers, as appears in the initial healing phase of a tendon or ligament injury, has random fiber orientation. Consequently, only a small proportion of the fibers have the proper alignment to carry any tension load applied to the scar, and the resulting scar exhibits mechanical weakness. This probably explains the broadening of surgical scars located where significant distraction forces act on the wound edges. *Right:* In a spatially ordered and aligned mass of fibers (as one finds in normal tendon, ligament, and fascia, and as exists at the end of the remodeling phase of wound scars), all fibers carry a tension load, so that the same mass of tissue exhibits more than a three-fold increase in strength and rigidity, provided of course that the load aligns parallel to those fibers.

the latter represent a minor fraction of the total collagen mass, that mass as an entity exhibits quite poor tensile strength and rigidity.

The material in two preceding sections can be expressed in the form of a word diagram to crystallize the nature of the cause-effect sequences and in formational flow. Thus, the following:

FIBROUS TISSUE REPAIR

(Injury) → *(Fibrous tissue)* → *(Scar)* → *(Replacement)*
↑
(Mechanical forces)

I assume (lacking direct proof for the idea or to the contrary) that the callus remodeling process just described results from some physical-chemical property of the fibrous tissue such that when a tension load overstretches it, it generates and delivers to the cells contained within it an activating stimulus that leads to proliferation of the mesenchymal cells and the production thereby of new differentiated cells. Some of these cells must remove "packets" of the preexisting scar (we might term them "fibroclasts"), and others (the fibroblasts) then replace it with new collagen which deposits in parallel alignment with the tension loads in the region. Since the tropocollagen molecules seem to polymerize outside the cells that made them, it would most likely constitute microenvironmental (as R. Young puts it) physicochemical factors that determine the spatial orientation of the polymer structure. This replacement sequence strongly resembles the manner in which the initial bony fracture callus eventually becomes wholly replaced by mature lamellar bone.

Normal Remodeling of Mature Fibrous Tissue

Little has been written of such a phenomenon, and some students of such matters have categorically denied that it occurs, possibly because little convincing evidence of it has appeared in studies of collagen turnover in the mouse and rat. (For a lead into the current status of our experimental knowledge of this problem, see Klein *et al.*⁵⁴)

However, clinical evidence convinces me that remodeling, used in the sense of a normal slow rate of turnover of the tissue, mediated by the activity of differentiated cells, does occur in most—if not all—fibrous tissue organs in man. Since my clinical evidence belongs in the circumstantial rather than in the proof category, the doubting reader may feel perfectly free to take issue with the following remarks.

Several facts seem pertinent to this particular argument. *First,* spontaneous tendon and ligament ruptures occur very rarely when expressed as failures per number of tension load-deload events in the general population at any age (as already noted, well below 1/100,000,000 failure/cycles). *Second,* no nonviable structural material known, whether organic or inorganic, natural or man-made, displays immunity to failure in mechanical fatigue. The *relative* immunity exhibited by bone and fibrous tissue in life depends upon their intrinsic viability; when infarcted by some means (such as by free grafting) but left in the body to carry mechanical loads, both lose their immunity to fatigue and do not regain it until after some months have passed. During that time, and if mechanically unprotected, a bone graft can break or a tendon or ligament graft elongate hopelessly. I would argue here that this susceptible period represents the time required for adequate revascularization and repopulation of the structure by biomechanically competent lines of cells.

Third, when one of the rare spontaneous ruptures of fibrous tissues organs does occur, it usually happens after age 30, not before, which suggests a time-dependent fatigue-like process (just yesterday I repaired one in the posterior tibial tendon of a 55-year-old man). If it takes so long for such a process to become manifest, one can easily understand why similar failures remain practically unknown in animal species such as the chicken, rat, rabbit, and dog; their natural lifespans end long before it can happen. *Fourth,* while microscopic sections of healthy fibrous tissue organs rarely show regions of cellular activity that suggest a turnover process such as already described, *nevertheless they do show them* and with about the same frequency (or rarity if you prefer) per unit volume of tissue as one finds active bone remodeling centers in the compacta of healthy people in the same age range. This means something in the order of two remodeling processes annually per cubic millimeter of tendon or ligament.

I infer from these facts that in normal human adults turnover (i.e. remodeling) of fibrous tissue organs regularly takes place, and that the annual fraction of the tissue turned over approximates that in human cortical bone, approximately one per cent to five per cent per year. I infer too that this turnover has a particular and major biomechanical function: It replaces small regions of mechanical fatigue-like damage with new and mechanically undamaged collagenous tissue. Such a mechanism would make an intact fibrous tissue *organ* practically immune to gross structural fatigue failure even though its *material* is not immune in the microscopic sense, exactly what we observe and seek to explain.

Disease of the Remodeling Mechanism

Finally, I infer and propose that some impairment in the fibrous tissue remodeling process causes most of the "spontaneous" ruptures of tendons and ligaments which we do see in otherwise healthy people. The obvious evidence of degeneration one finds in the tendon ends at operation of a fresh one suggest that. The degeneration has consistently attained naked-eye visibility, and microscopic sections of a biopsy of the freshly ruptured ends consistently confirm it. This discussion excludes local disease processes which provide obvious and specific other underlying causes of such weakening and/or degeneration, for example rheumatoid synovitis or rubbing of a tendon over a postfracture bony irregularity.

WHY AND HOW?

What effects of tensile loading activates the cells in fibrous tissue, and what causes differentiation of new cells into fibroblasts (rather than into osteoblasts or even lipoblasts)? Are those

182   *The Physiology of Cartilaginous, Fibrous, and Bony Tissue*

effects essentially physical, chemical, biological, or some combination?

What causes the collagen fibers, as they polymerize outside the cell, to align parallel to the tension resultant: some physicochemical effect or a biological one?

How much stretch, how often, how quickly applied, of what duration accounts for the Stretch-Hypertrophy Law?

The above form some of the important questions for research in this area in the coming years.

QUESTIONS

According to the proposals of this text:
1. What determines a tendon's and ligament's diameter?
2. What determines the thickness of a sheet of fascia? Therefore, finding a very tenuous fascia in an anatomical location where one normally might find a thick one probably means what?
3. What determines the strength of the plantar fascia? In what respect does any tendency of it to fatigue as a device supporting the longitudinal arch of the foot differ from the fatigue experienced by the muscles that help to support that arch?
4. What (probably) makes normal fibrous tissues immune to mechanical fatigue failures, and what for bone?
5. You are operating to lengthen (and thus weaken) the posterior tibial tendon in a child with severe spastic forefoot adductus and heel varus. You find the posterior tibial tendon no larger in diameter than one of the long digital flexor or extensor tendons. What does that mean? What should you do?
6. Why (probably) do free ligament grafts and many free tendon grafts fail by stretching out? How could you change your plan of management to compensate for it and thereby increase your fraction of successes?

Aphorism

Mustof's Disease

Let me here introduce you to this purely clinical entity, well and long known to competent clinicians but not until now digni-

Biomechanical Response Characteristics of Fibrous Tissue 183

fied by a unique cognomen. I do so partly for general educational purposes and partly because it relates rather directly to material in the next two chapters. An actual example will convey the message with adequate clarity.

A 17-year-old girl came to the emergency room complaining of pain in her wrist of two weeks or so duration, which she attributed to a fall. Examination revealed diffuse tenderness and swelling; x-rays appeared normal. She was told she sprained it and to bandage it and apply warm soaks. She returned five days later with the same complaints and findings and so was placed in a volar plaster mold and the earlier advice reemphasized. She returned again five days later with the same complaints and findings and so was placed in a short arm cast and lectured—gently, though—on making mountains out of anthills. She returned again after ten more days with the same complaints. At this juncture the Emergency Room physician called our clinic and asked if we could help him to handle and "pacify" this difficult patient.

We removed the cast and found a wrist that was swollen, warm, diffusely tender, and very painful on motion.

What would you do at this juncture?

Drs. Wallace Johnson and Anthony Majestro and I were impressed by the fact that when immobilized in plaster, true sprains rapidly cease hurting and their swelling subsides; this young lady's wrist had not done so, a very simple but, in terms of its diagnostic implications, very meaningful inconsistency. It in effect waved a red flag before our eyes imprinted with the words "does not compute." We inquired about the so-called "sprain" in some detail and discovered therefrom that she had no true recollection of any such incident but, because the wrist began to hurt, she simply had assumed she "must of" (hence, *Mustof's*) fallen on it, and she had relayed that to the initial physician who, under pressure to work through a large patient load, did not question it.

We ordered a new x-ray, which revealed marked narrowing of the carpal joint spaces. Further studies revealed this to have been a pyarthrosis of the wrist.

Thus, "Mustof's" disease, which represents a falsely conceived cause-effect relation that can lead to serious errors in diagnosis and treatment. Most such errors have their origin, not in faulty erudition or out of ignorance of the literature and basic medical sciences, but rather in the strategy one follows in obtaining information to add up. The following chapter deals with an analogous problem in orthopaedic basic research, and with one means of minimizing its effects on our research productivity.

I believe that in time the proposed solution can be adapted to the problem of clinical diagnosis, which is why it appears in such a book as this.

Chapter IX

An Optimizing Strategy for Medical Research

Serendipity, while sometimes a dazzling contender, in the long run leads very inefficiently and slowly towards mastery of human disease. Our own inherent biases have distorted the output of the logical process in past attempts to devise something better. Probability and cause-effect properties, now known to characterize all living organisms, permit one to study disease in ways which can enhance greatly over pure chance the probability that such study will succeed.

Using such features of biological systems, this chapter builds a simple strategy which does exactly that.

In mastering human disease, a two-stage process, one must first identify the cause of disease and then learn how to understand and control it; the strategy in this chapter applies primarily to the former activity.

INTRODUCTION*

This chapter proposes to scientists engaged in and persons responsible for guiding and funding our orthopaedic medical research a strategy or algorithm which might improve, possibly very greatly, their productivity by increasing not their volume but rather the *probable relevance* (1)** of their data to a particular basic goal of medical research, a goal we will define shortly.

A phenomenon encountered in medical education (and delineated in the preceding aphorism) first exposed the kernel of this problem to me, and since it still exists abundantly there and in

---

*This constitutes an edited version of a paper first read by the author at the University of Guelph Veterinary College at Guelph, Ontario, Canada, March 1969, and of another currently in press in a symposium volume edited by Professor W. S. S. Jee and published by the University of Utah Press.

**The numbers in parentheses signify explanatory notes found at the end of this chapter.

medical research also, and since it relates closely to the present subject, I will describe it next.

For over 20 years I have helped to train orthopaedic surgeons, an effort which attempts to develop in them the ability to make correct and perceptive diagnoses and to choose correct treatments. During that activity those trainees demonstrated, both repeatedly and consistently, a little acknowledged property of diagnostic and therapeutic errors, to wit: *Most such errors directly follow decisions based upon trivial and/or incomplete facts.*

> *Nota bene:* Poor scholarship or mediocre intelligence per se cause only a minor fraction of those errors, although inexperienced clinicians often attribute them more to such causes than to any activities in the clinical "action" which, as it were, set the stage for a proper exercise of scholarship. Most teachers in medicine see often enough the scholastically able and even brilliant man who nevertheless consistently makes more clinical mistakes (i.e. turns up more instances of Mustof's disease) than some of his less erudite colleagues.

Even in extremely taxing medical problems, the final lists of relevant facts arrayed in order of real importance repeatedly are short and allow most fourth-year medical students to suggest the correct diagnoses. This contrasts strongly with the equally repeated fact that widely experienced and very astute clinicians might have worked long and very hard to obtain the evidence needed to construct those lists. These circumstances point not to poor scholarly talent but to something else associated with actual performance and with the very process of obtaining basic working information relevant to a given problem as the cause of most clinical errors.* Feinstein recently voiced a similar view although he phrased it in other words.[28]

Present-day medical education still lacks totally any formalized, codified strategy for teaching these prescholarship mental skills, as I call them, and in cognizance of that tends to substitute performing complete histories and physical examinations on every

---

*Curiously, most of my friends actively engaged in the private practice of medicine recognize the truth and impact of this statement immediately but many of my friends in Academia find it puzzling, or even disturbing.

patient and mastering the literature of all the special fields in medicine. Yet, in a society with a doctor shortage that substitute would cause real disaster, for while waiting for physicians to complete examining patients with bruised fingers or minor skin rashes, other patients would die of myocardial infarcts or appendicitis.

Plainly, when too few doctors exist to satisfy the total need, *one must establish priorities* to minimize sacrificing the very ill by diverting medical expertise to trivial problems. Many of my own early teachers—J. W. O'Meara of Worcester (deceased); F. N. Potts (deceased), G. Marcy, B. Obletz, R. Payne, J. D. Godfrey, and R. Erickson, all of Buffalo; and B. Andrews of Worcester (deceased)—are (or were) very good surgeons, not because they achieved eminence in a basic science but exactly because they learned how to assign clinical priorities wisely.

The same priority problem would exist in research if too few investigators and insufficient funds and facilities existed to fulfill the need. And that is precisely true.

As a resident some 24 years ago that priority problem confronted me; later I found (and still find) its parallel abundantly present in medical research. While that led to a search for some way to enhance the quality of my own research sufficiently to gain a paid trip to Stockholm, I soon realized (along with the truly great improbability of ever taking that particular trip) that no such strategy was available, at least in any form that could serve questing young physicians. Even today that holds true, so that effective and competent medical practice as well as research often appear to neophytes more as occult arts than exact sciences. Let us crystallize the kernel of the above material at this juncture: *In both clinical medicine and medical research, the tactics of data acquisition often lack effective strategic direction.*

What does that mean?—That a poorly conceived strategy can deploy research at its very inception so as to almost ensure that it will not achieve its goal. Often we win battles while losing wars; or we drive exquisitely designed racing cars up dead-end, curving, boulder-strewn dirt roads.

The above realizations gelled rather slowly, but if you can

accept them, they lead directly to the following axiomatic realizations:

1. Obtaining data, clearly a distinct part of the investigative process (and here arbitrarily termed a tactical one), must transpire *before* one has exactly the right data to interpret and analyze; otherwise one needs no research, for having the right data transforms the matter from a search into the unknown into understanding the known.

2. The true relevance of research data to the basic research goal limits its content of information about that goal, and no matter how brilliant the analyst he cannot extract more intelligence about that goal than his data actually contain (2).

3. Clearly, then, the way one deploys his initial fact-finding endeavors must affect that relevance and also the speed with which he reaches the heart of the matter.

While the problem of how to analyze data already on hand has received considerable formal attention and a few persons have even recognized data acquisition as a separate, prior, and important strategic problem (Feinstein,[28] Polanyi[71]), I know of no formulation of an effective and general *data acquisition strategy* for use in goal-oriented medical research. After all, could one really contrive such a thing? Categorically, I say yes, based in part upon probability considerations, in part upon the current level of development of biological knowledge of which we make relatively inefficient use, and in part upon its demonstrated actual effect on work in my own laboratory. This text summarizes it.

A GOAL FOR MEDICAL RESEARCH

Goal and strategy relate in research as heads to tails in coins; furthermore, the nature of the goal establishes what will prove effective and ineffective in terms of strategy. So, at this juncture let us identify a basic goal of most medical research, the particular one to which my own research and this chapter have been addressed. That we can do quickly, for here medical experience and wisdom speak clearly, briefly, and bluntly.

An Optimizing Strategy for Medical Research 189

For each patient we truly cure (*not* the same thing as treat), ignorance about our body frustrates efforts to cure many dozens of others (Ambrose Paré said it well: "I dress wounds; God heals them"). Exactly that frustration, so repeatedly encountered in any clinic or medical office, makes most physicians search for and (like our patients, whose taxes fund much of our medical research) assign very high value to *accurate* and *reliable* ways of *diagnosing, preventing,* and *curing* disease.

For brevity, let the term "systems control capability" designate those abilities. Exactly that goal underlies most medical research (2), *and only in that context does the remaining text apply.* Should some readers find that definition redundant, try a little game I have played over the years: In series, ask the next 10 colleagues you meet their concept of the basic goal of medical research. The vagueness and marginal relevance of the responses may surprise you.

ORGANIZATIONAL PROPERTIES OF BIOLOGICAL SYSTEMS

Given a goal for medical research in the broad sense, let us next define and describe a few simple and well-known properties of biological systems in a way and with emphases which can serve us later in the strategic sense. First then, four simple definitions.

Definitions

System: Any collection of two or more things which mutually interact form a system. A subclass of *real* systems (i.e. those natural and artificial systems made of matter) could include physical, mechanical, biological, electronic, and chemical complexes. A subclass of *abstract* systems (which contain no matter) could include calculus, thermodynamics, music, economic theory, and Kant. In relation to human perception, experience, objectives, and thought, any system may exhibit *purposeful* behavior or the contrary. The subsequent discussion will deal with the human body, a good example of a real purposeful system.

Properties signify any and all catalogable facts about a system, whether important or trivial, simple or complex, real or abstract.

Functions signify those few properties which determine a system's optimal purposeful performance in, and its interaction with, its environment. Thus, functions form a subset of the universal set of properties. In addition to first, second, and higher-order meanings, note that functions also have a relative connotation. For example, inability to oppose the thumb forms a disability in a man but we consider it normal in a monkey. And hemoglobin S potentiates human survival in those parts of the world where malaria exists endemically but can cause serious disease in malaria-free cultures and climates.

Trivia signify all nonfunctional properties (i.e. the complement of the functional subset); furthermore, and very important strategically, *trivia vastly outnumber functions* in all biological systems, or, as a kind of verbal equation:

EQUATION 13

$$Properties = Functions + trivia$$
$$(Functions < trivia)$$

Now let us describe selected properties.

Properties of the Organization of the Human Body

Interaction forms the essence of any function (3). One class of such interactions occurs between the system and its external environment; a second class, subservient to the needs of the first, occurs within the system. For example, one function of bone consists of supplying in a particular spatial orientation a rigid support against which muscles can pull. A bone dissected free of those muscles no longer provides that function, *and therefore one cannot study that function in such a preparation.* The interaction which represents its essence has been destroyed. While one certainly can study mechanical strength as well as material properties in such a preparation, those properties alone do not represent its function in the body (3).

We might write this as another verbal equation, thus:

EQUATION 14

(Properties of Bone) ⇌ (Properties of Muscle)

> *Nota bene:* The arrows indicating the interaction represent the first-order functions. Specifically, the bone or the muscle alone do not *and cannot.* This point may seem subtle to some and ridiculous to others but nevertheless it is real and of fundamental nature; ignoring it will affect, and devastatingly so, the goal-oriented value of any research.

Another example: The parathyroid glands produce a hormone in response to fluctuations in the serum calcium ion concentration. The function or purpose of that production we believe consists of maintaining the serum ionized calcium within marrow limits. The essential interactions constituting that function occur only partly between the blood and the gland. Partly they occur at all of the other blood-body interfaces at which parathormone can act to alter serum ionized calcium. Or, as a word equation:

EQUATION 15

(Parathyroid gland) ⇌ $\overline{Blood}$ ⇌ Body

Thus, the blood may simply act as a cause-effect relay, connecting the parathyroid gland in meaningful ways (i.e. allowing it to interact with) the gut, kidney, bone marrow, bone, and possibly other systems.* Such interactions do not exist in *in vitro* preparations of the gland.

One cannot, therefore, study parathyroid *functions* by studying its glandular tissue in isolated cell-culture or organ-culture systems; instead, such isolated systems allow one to study the tissue's *properties.* Lacking positive foreknowledge (i.e. prior and accurate identification) of which among its thousands of innumerable

---

*Clinical experience has convinced me that it does interact with some other system, unknown so far as to its identity.

192 *The Physiology of Cartilaginous, Fibrous, and Bony Tissue*

properties participate essentially in its few functions (recall here that trivial properties *vastly* outnumber functional ones and that functions represent *interactions*), and lacking foreknowledge of how they do so, such *ex vivo* study has very low probability of producing data *relevant to any real disease* of the system (1). That is the rub: Such systems easily produce very large volumes of data, but not so easily can one ensure the relevance of those data to the basic goal defined in this chapter.

Organization of function exists in all such systems, i.e. their internal anatomical and cause-effect relationships exhibit meaningful structure, and in both the vertical and horizontal senses. Thus, separate levels or layers of functional organization exist, and each level has separate coexisting categories. Note here that mere visual perception of the morphological organization of a biological system can befog one's perception of the nature and the organization of the functions it primarily exists to provide and/or subserve.

Two additional real properties of biological systems, derived from the nature of the biological organization just mentioned, play a very important role in developing this strategy.

The Dendritic Property

A root-like structure characterizes the cause-effect trajectories which connect the functions of an intact man to their macromolecular level basis. As a result, any one identifiable function (or disease) of the intact man has thousands of possible underlying macromolecular-level determinants. Well-structured and exactly identifiable *chains of cause-effect interactions* (usually greatly restricted in number relative to the theoretically possible total) lead downwards, in step-by-step fashion, from the intact man to each macromolecule. While in this scheme of organization *all upwards routes converge* towards the common locus of the intact man, the branching routes *diverge downwards*, leading to many thousands of individual macromolecular-level properties. As we shall see shortly, this has the effect that simply *finding* the one macromolecular aberration that causes a disease in its biological surroundings of thousands of noncausal macromolecules, properties, and interactions resembles the problem of finding a needle in a haystack and also the "20 Questions" game once popular on television (4).

The dendritic property causes analyses of physiological systems which proceed *downwards* through increasingly elementary levels of internal organization to have a far greater *probability* of identifying within any finite time period the macromolecular determinants of a disease or function than do analyses which start at the bottom level and proceed *upwards* (6). This statistical— and potentially controversial (5)— property deserves special emphasis and treatment; Figure 9.01 accords it this by depicting the dendritic cause-effect "tree" which characterizes all natural, purposeful systems.

In addition to the dendritic property, another organizational property becomes relevant here, as follows.

The Associative Property

As Polanyi[71] and Mayr[64] observed in different ways, when two or more elementary building blocks (such as cells) associate in particular ways to create new kinds of systems building blocks at higher levels of organization (such as a renal nephron, a lung alveolus, or a bone BMU), *new functions emerge at the higher level which belong uniquely to the association,* i.e. they have no analog in lower level elements. Example: Countercurrent flow exists in the nephron but not in any single one of its cells.

Downwards analyses of biological systems can now readily and efficiently *identify* such functions, but knowledge only of a system's atomistic properties never permits one to identify them, nor even to predict them with any useful probability (6). For example, one could no more identify or predict the structure and purpose of a kidney by studying only its cells than he could the structure and purpose of a steering wheel by studying the physics of the iron atoms or crystals composing it.

Other Examples: No single cell loves, ponders its origins and ultimate fate, or distinguishes beauty from ugliness, but the cellular association named "man" does.

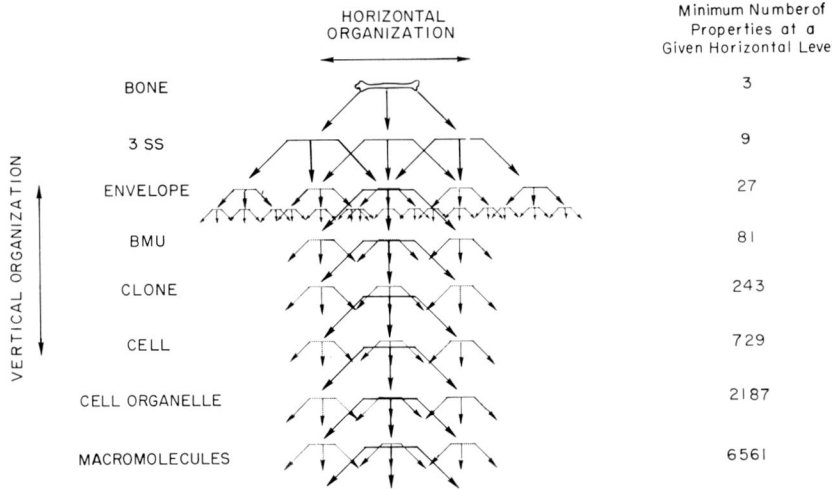

Figure 9.01. The dendritic property of cause-effect in biological organization. Assume that only three subsystems completely determine the properties of a bone, and each of them in turn depends solely on only three sub-subsystems for all of its properties, and so on down to macromolecules. Then, given the seven presently known vertical levels of organization in bone as an organ, more than 6,500 macromolecular niduses exist which might cause a disease. Assume further a particular disease, say osteogenesis imperfecta, which has one macromolecular cause. Which forms the most efficient search strategy in trying to identify it: Begin at the bottom, or at the top?

To achieve probability 0.5 of finding it by studying the macromolecular properties, one would have to study *completely* more than 3,500 of them, i.e. he must make 3,500 moves—a problem of enormous magnitude. By proceeding downwards, he would locate it *in only seven moves.* That represents a more than 900-fold enhancement in search efficiency and speed, and I have deliberately understated the argument; in reality it probably exceeds 1000-fold.

A well encompasses a body of fluid, which no single one of its stones can do.

No theft, rape, riot, or murder exist in a world containing only one human being. In each above instance, knowledge of the intact system, not of its atomistic elements, taught us these things; in each of them, interaction introduced something new and not present in the individual atomistic members.

Disease in biological systems signifies malfunction, or, if you prefer, defective purposeful behavior, and so arises from one or more disturbed functions. According to this viewpoint, function and disease represent opposite faces of the same coin; then, and since function can be relative, disease must be also. Example: A congenital inability to create bone, lethal for man, occurs quite normally in sharks. (*Note:* By definition a trivial abnormality does not cause disease, while an abnormal function does.)

HAYSTACK LOGISTICS

Let us now draw two strategically helpful parallels from outside of the biological sciences.

Excepting things such as stab wounds, boyish gastronomic excesses, and thermal burns, the underlying causes of human disease usually lie at low levels of organization in the system and represent either single, or a combination of a relatively few, individual defects. Many thousands of kinds of macromolecules exist even in a single cell, however, and many thousands more interactions exist between them, both individually and in the forms of organized associations. As a logistic problem, then: *Finding the ultimate cause of a disease* (such as diabetes, gout, or "marble bone" disease) *resembles finding a needle in a haystack.*

Were one to approach the real needle-in-a-haystack problem by patiently sorting out by hand the entire haystack, with high probability two things would ensue: It would take a *very* long time to find the needle; furthermore, a high and separate conditioning probability would exist of overlooking the needle when ultimately the sorting hand approached it. Consequently, from its very inception the odds stack heavily against success within any reasonable period of time and amount of effort when one chooses such a strategy. *As an identification mechanism*, a sensitive magnetometer would greatly enhance the accuracy of such a search by greatly reducing the separate probability of overlooking the needle. An *efficient search strategy*, serving to deploy the use of the magnetometer, could enhance the *speed* of that search without impairing its accuracy.

In regard to search strategy, consider briefly the strategically helpful "20 Questions" problem or game as it was once played on television. In this game, a panel tries to identify a single fact unknown to them and selected from all other cataloged knowledge that, *for the purpose of that moment,* has become irrelevant. Furthermore, the panel must do so by asking the quizzee up to 20 questions, each answerable only by "yes" or "no." (The yes or no answer analogizes the magnetometer, which in effect says the needle does lie in that mass of hay or it does not.) Obviously, were one to try to succeed by beginning to enumerate all facts in random order, he would not live long enough to succeed once, even if he played the game all day and all night until he died. This is simply the haystack problem again but with an added quirk which makes a critical issue of the search strategy matter: One must find the needle in 20 "moves" or less.

A consistent level of success within the allotted 20 questions therefore demands some kind of search strategy which *enormously* improves the odds of success over random enumeration of individual facts. While some of my scientific contemporaries may take offense at the implication that much medical research suffers from an analogously silly strategic deployment, I will risk that offense because I firmly believe it does. The players of the 20 Questions game evolved exactly such a strategy, and it had two basic and really quite simple elements.

First, they organized all knowledge into vertical and horizontal categories and subcategories, such that a *dendritic chain* of downwardly branching nature connected all possible individual facts to the universal collection of facts, an abstract structure which strikingly resembles the basic dendritic cause-effect structure found in the organization of physiological systems.

Second, the players then "searched" through the dendritic loci in that atlas. (Each intersection or junction of a branching path represented a cleavage of facts into two groups, just like breaking a mass of hay into two halves.) They did so *by starting at the top level* (example: Is it biological or mineral?) and then proceeded level-by-level downwards (If biological, is it living or dead?) in binary steps through increasingly specific and restricted layers and categories of information. With a little psychology and ingenuity they often got far more than one "bit" of information per question. This strategy did indeed enormously enhance the probability of *identifying* within the limits of their resources (for them, 20 questions; for you and me, our annual grant funds and the limiting patience of those who dispense them) the one relevant fact among the multiple millions of, for the purpose of the moment, irrelevant or trivial ones. I can say categorically that it did so because in point of fact the real players won that game more often than not.

The answers of the quizzees to their questions provide the analog of the haystack magnetometer as previously noted; *their questioning pattern constituted a search strategy for deploying it;* their atlas of knowledge permitted that search strategy to possess high efficiency, and, in point of stochastic fact, nearly the maximum possible efficiency in terms of the number of questions or moves made.

I propose a closely analogous strategy for our orthopaedic basic research into unknown systems (4) as outlined next, quite as simple in its essence as it differs from much contemporary research practice.

STRATEGIC CONSIDERATIONS

To repeat (because other aims have legitimate existence): *Granted a systems control capability goal,* the following occurs:

1. If purposeful *behavior* constitutes a system's functional essence, then you should focus on it. In that case, mastering an unknown system (an unknown system here designates one whose behavior you cannot control well enough to suit your purposes and needs (4)) requires searching for, identifying, and then understanding its behavioral elements as well as their sum; that includes especially the underlying *cause-effect interactions* which form the system's collection of functions.

Note: Anatomy and form, from the gross to the electron microscopic level, chemical and physical composition, or epidemiology and the like must serve here not as ends unto themselves but as *means to identify and/or to study behavior.* One certainly would not deny their study as ends unto themselves to those so inclined (science forms a large fabric with many and diverse regions); rather, let us hope that those who allocate grant funds should choose such investigations with some larger strategy in mind, so that many separate projects give some promise of fitting into some medically utilitarian whole.

2. Studying trivia wastes valuable research resources, and trivia do not always—or even usually—make themselves self-evident; reflect on the enormous literature which, 10 or more years after publication, proved to deal with trivia from a control system capability viewpoint. While admitting freely the arbitrary nature of that viewpoint, I must insist *on the basis of every incurable patient physicians see* that it constitutes a perfectly valid and proper one for investigators and granting agencies.

Inasmuch as trivia greatly outnumber functions in all biological systems (in fact, probably by more than 1000:1), choosing a subject to study by some random process (7) will, with probability exceeding .999, cause it and its study to prove trivial, that is, wasteful. No sane investigator would invest effort on such abysmally poor odds were he satisfied that much better ones were available.

3. So, to increase the probability of studying true functions we need some way to improve the accuracy with which we *identify* them and distinguish them from trivia, i.e. we need a research analog of the magnetometer in the haystack problem. A simple, highly effective analog consists of *comparing diseased to normal states,* as Johnson[53] among others has pointed out. In a disease a malfunction assuredly exists, and its location in the system should appear as a telltale and characteristic difference from the healthy state. Finding it then becomes a matter of locating the right difference, which one does by making the right comparison.

Now, in looking for that comparison, we can adapt the "20 Questions" strategy or *search pattern* to the biological problem, enhancing the probability that we will identify the causal malfunction (this time a biological needle in a physiological haystack) before we exhaust our limited resources in the effort. The following two-element strategem can achieve that.

4. *The Systems Atlas: First,* one needs some scheme which organizes all meaningful information about the system's physiology into realistic, dendritically structured vertical levels and horizontal categories, just as the television panel did with a far more inclusive body of information. I will call such a scheme a "systems atlas" henceforth, a term you may recall from earlier figures in this volume.

To crystallize previous material as it bears on this matter, this atlas should (a) *identify* the system's functions, which effective comparison of normal to diseased states can serve to expedite (this requires an extensive and viable descriptive catalog of such states, so that pure description has considerable value in this scheme), and (b) simultaneously *map* the cause-effect dendritic chains which lead from the physiological functions of the intact man downwards towards their macromolecular level determinants. In one view these chains constitute the routes of normal communication and regulation within the system, and in another view but at the same time they provide one means to specify all of its possible internal malfunctions.

If at some particular frontier of physiological organization no such atlas exists, then constructing one should receive topmost priority in the overall planning of research into it. This does not constitute as trivial a matter as some may think; as examples, in the light of the "unknown" test referred to above (4), we do not yet understand the brain, the skeleton, the body's articulations, neoplasia, aging, atherosclerotic vascular disease, renal failure, or hepatic cirrhosis, for we cannot yet cure even one per cent of the malfunctions of such systems by our own active and rational intervention. Even wounds heal by themselves; in 6000 years of working on that problem we have learned many things *not* to do because they impede it but none yet that evoke it in response to movements of our own baton.

Second, given at least a first approximation of a systems atlas for one of the body's systems, then begin to study one or more of its diseases by searching through the known part of the atlas' structure, proceeding downwards through progressively more elementary levels, to *identify* the ultimate cause of the disease in its surround of (for the purposes of understanding any one disease) trivial "noise." Obviously, given some initial headway on the atlas, one can then begin to use it in the study of some particular disease. Thus, both efforts can proceed together, although the degree of development of the atlas must always "lead" the effective study of any disease.

Third, then try to *understand* these causes, a problem beyond the scope of this argument and one which often affords molecular biology its ideal tactical field of exercise.

> *Nota bene:* One needs some objective way to determine when research planned as above has succeeded in the overall and collective sense. Such success could constitute the ability to diagnose, prevent, and/or cure some given percentage of those persons in our country who have any disease. Obviously, we must establish the numerical value of such a percentage on a purely arbitrary basis, for no natural level of systems control capability exists to my knowledge, and becoming able to cure everything, like perfection, probably remains an unattainable goal even over the next millenium (8).

Fourth, I have implied several times before and now state categorically that *identifying* a problem and then *understanding* it form totally different investigative challenges which usually require different tactical approaches (and even different investigator psychology and kinds of intellectual talents).

Fifth, a matter not previously mentioned herein: One must design his initial approach to an unknown system with what ultimately proves fragmentary and often actually inappropriate (i.e. trivial) information. These things become evident as the work progresses, so common sense requires that one periodically evaluate past progress in order to change goals, strategy, and/or tactics as proves necessary to maintain an optimum probability of success of the work. Thus, rigid minds cannot plough such fields; they nurture only the flexible and versatile. Rigid minds soon get their plows hopelessly stuck on a rock or stump, where flexible ones simply bypass them.

COMMENT

Applying the preceding ideas to an actual biological system will illustrate at least partially their practical use. Briefly, the next chapter will sketch the beginning of a systems atlas of bone and then illustrate with two skeletal problems how its use significantly advanced our understanding of them. The initial step in the above strategy, the construction of a systems atlas of the human skeleton, has occupied most of my own research effort for two decades and, as spin off, led to the publications listed among the initial pages of this book.

The strategic development of skeletal physiology remains fragmentary, for the strategic moves abstracted here and in subsequent volumes of this series deal only, and still incompletely, with the remodeling and modeling cellular subsystems. Endochondral ossification, the repair mechanisms which pertain to each of these three major subsystems, and the skeletal roles in calcium, electrolyte, and acid-base homeostasis pose operationally distinct problems of their own and require analogous strategic development in the future. Until we achieve it, our skeletal diagnostic capability will remain empirical, largely descriptive, and relatively unperceptive. Only after its development can we hope to approach with reasonable expectations of large-scale, rapid, and consistent success the problems of preventing and curing most of the entities which a perceptive diagnostic capability can identify.

A serious possibility exists in my mind that the strategy proposed herein could also materially accelerate acquiring better understanding of today's troublesome and erratically behaving social, ecological, and political systems if we made an effort to apply it systematically in interpreting research findings, in conceiving and designing observations and experiments, and in formulating grant support policy. I have some reservations about our capacity to augment in like proportion how wisely we might use any such improved expertise, reservations based on man's demonstrated proclivity for bending his technological and scientific advances simultaneously to both constructive and destructive ends, and at both the individual and collective levels of social organization.

NOTES

1. An obvious example of what "relevance" signifies here: Assume one must *identify* the computer-oriented function of an electronic computer module; if he chose to do so by analyzing its chemical composition almost certainly he would fail, for that composition has very low relevance indeed to the study's goal (although it could help to understand how it supplied its function, *after identification of the function*. No matter how complete the information eventually obtained about its chemical composition, its very nature or relevance will restrict the insight it can provide into the computer-oriented role of the device.

2. I just left a charming and courageous young lady whose thin, fragile bones have undergone numerous fractures and have hideously and irreparably deformed her. She has osteogenesis imperfecta, or brittle bones, a congenital bone disease for which we lack any cure. (Incidentally, a tentative study of that problem in our laboratory according to this strategy revealed clearly why all past efforts to understand it failed; they took the wrong dendrite in the systems atlas. That study did also point out the correct dendrite or, if you prefer, cause-effect trajectory. See A. R. Villanueva and H. M. Frost, *Acta Scand Orthop 41*:531, 1970.) She knows that her deformities as well as her blighted germ plasm will deny her most of the normal joys and fulfillments of womanhood; her parents' expressions reveal a parallel perceptiveness, plus the pain of watching helplessly a tragedy personified in one's own child. Such situations instill an unashamed utilitarian, goal-oriented, control-capability purpose, as well as persistence into most physicians' research.

3. Three arithmetic calculators can have identical computational potential, yet one may consist of an assemblage of electronic components, another of purely mechanical parts, and a third of

the cells of the human brain. These examples illustrate a basic point: In systems a specific function represents a particular *behavioral relation* (or *interaction*) between two or more things but never a static single physical fact or property which can retain its identity and functional essence in a state of total isolation from the remainder of the system.

4. Here an "unknown" system signifies *any over which we lack a reliable systems control capability.* A familar name (brain) and recognition of certain organ-level functions (cerebrate, compute, emote, compare, evaluate; or id, superego) do not dig deeply enough into the functional stuffing of a system to show us how to control its malfunctions. By such a standard the brain forms an unknown system, for we cannot cure consistently and by intentional actions the psychopath, the thief, the bigot, the child beater, the liar.

5. One controversial potential in this statement lies in the emotional reaction to it of some molecular biologists, for in effect I say that, as holds true for the rest of us "nonmolecular" biologists, they work in a field which forms only another and small part of the elephant of knowledge, not one of its major and certainly not one of its self-sufficient fractions.

6. Probability considerations make this impractical. Consider, for example, a brain with 10^{10} possible neuronal associations and states. Lacking detailed knowledge of the brain's actual functional structure as well as identification of all of its internal intermediate-level functions, the statistical probability differs negligibly from zero that by randomly combining 10^{10} neurons in various ways 1000 scientists working continuously would, within any given 1000-year period, deliberately construct a device which duplicated the brain's actual functions, let alone its specific pattern of cellular associations and interactions.

Under such odds, it makes much better sense to try to find what already exists in nature than to try to predict it by *a priori* processes.

7. "Random" here means that no prior *proof* exists of a direct causal relation between the disease and the (randomly selected)

factor in question. While often we suspect a causal relation on the basis of observed *associations*, ultimately the vast majority of such inferences prove false and only the rare exceptions prove true, but, seemingly, only those do we remember later.

8. Practically speaking, a perfect control capability over a biological system would require an infinite expenditure of time, talent, and money, and so it represents an unattainable ideal. A feasible capability to strive for in medicine over the next 30 years would, from our present level of development and in my opinion, approximate the ability to diagnose and specify in terms of basic causes some 30 per cent of our diseases.

Chapter X

Application of Strategy

SYSTEMS ATLAS OF BONE

The first part of this chapter will outline the present degree of development of my own systems atlas of the neuromusculoskeletal system, one constructed much along the lines prescribed in the previous chapter and proven as valuable as hoped in use. Such use includes clinical analyses of skeletal disease—both reported and otherwise (Frame et al,[30, 31] Ramser et al,[73] Wu et al[102]) experimental design, and investigative strategy (Jee et al, [51, 52] Epker[27]). Following description of that atlas, the text will then briefly describe two specific situations in which its application led to new, unexpected, and valuable information.

Figure 10.01 diagrams the summed-up elements of this atlas along clinically oriented but strictly morphological lines. It does not look very promising, does it? Now, one could choose another basis than that for such a scheme and at least in principle could develop it into a very useful (but in principle not more, and equally not less, useful) atlas or instrument for directing research. For example, one could choose function as the chief foundation stone for such a basis, or even chemical processes, physical properties, or flow and usage of energy. Since my "thing" has constituted trying to identify function and match it with form, I will stay with it, observing that for clinicians like me it constitutes an easily understood and natural "feeling" scheme.

TABLE 10.01

ABBREVIATIONS IN CHAPTER X

BMU:	Basic multicellular unit of bone remodeling
ENOS:	Endochondral ossification
PMO:	Postmenopausal osteoporosis
3ss:	Triple surface system

206   *The Physiology of Cartilaginous, Fibrous, and Bony Tissue*

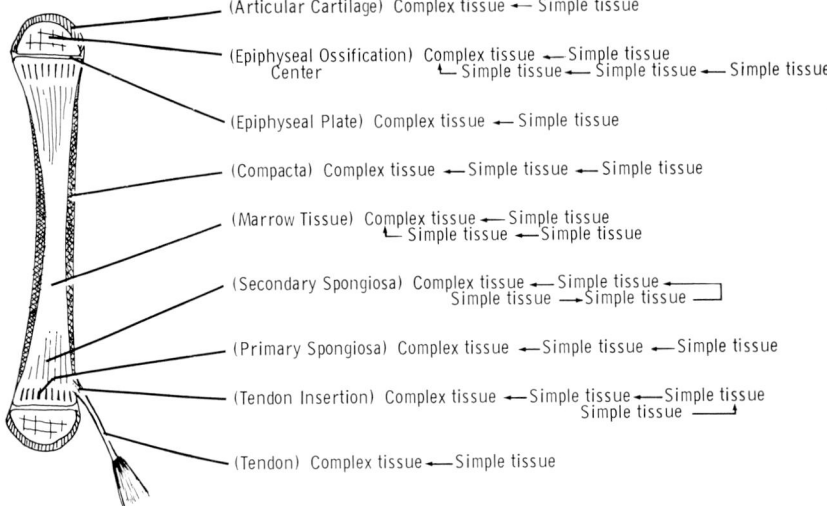

Figure 10.01. A diagram of an anatomical atlas or "compositional" map of a typical long bone as an organ, in which the inscriptions identify and name its various complex tissue components and lists for each one, without naming them, the corresponding number of simple tissue antecedents. For analytical purposes we can simplify considerably the problem of grasping all of this information; see Figure 10.02. For analytical purposes such a map is very hard to use.

We cannot here describe in detail each of the subsystems identified in Figure 10.01: it would be too time-consuming, space-consuming, and patience-taxing. So let us first present that material, arranged as morphologically named phenomena but now according to what we currently understand of cause-effect in the neuromusculoskeletal system. Figures 10.02 to 10.06 inclusive do this in the form of diagrams—the third time, incidentally, that I have attempted any such thing for the skeletal system. (First, reference 34; second, at Guelph, per the footnote at the beginning of the previous chapter.) To show how outside regulation of its activities relates to its cause-effect chains, Figure 10.06 provides a different "dimension" or view of this material.

Rather than outline all of the details shown in these five figures, I will simply illustrate the use of this systems atlas by developing only one of its downwardly branching dendritic paths, that which has proven to hold the keys to postmenopausal osteoporosis and to control of bone tissue turnover in human adults. That pathway will lead us to and below the compacta and should illustrate how one could dissect or analyze any other disease of the neuromuscular skeletal system. At this juncture then, inspect the figures mentioned and read their legends. You need not yet try to memorize them, for we will refer to them often in the text that follows.

The levels of organization between, including, and connecting an intact bone (the organ level in Fig. 10.02) to its macromolecular-level (and mostly cellularly based) activities include the following.

Organ Level

At this level lies the intact bone with all of its morphological properties and functions; we identified what I know of the latter in an earlier chapter. As Figures 10.01 and 10.02 imply, this is quite complicated—but only because of its numerous details; each detail is simple by itself and easily understood if isolated from the whole. Let us try to dissolve some of that seeming complexity by using some realistic simplifications and generalities to achieve such isolation.

Complex Tissue Level

Taken as an organ, a typical mature bone proves in the anatomical, biomechanical, and physiologic senses to represent the summed-up contributions of *only three groups of complex tissue histogenetic activities*, specifically those dependent upon endochondral ossification, those dependent on the histogenesis of compacta, and those of the fibrogenetic class. Figure 10.02 diagrams this.

Here the ENOS term will include all of its component complex tissues (articular and epiphyseal cartilage, primary and secondary

208   *The Physiology of Cartilaginous, Fibrous, and Bony Tissue*

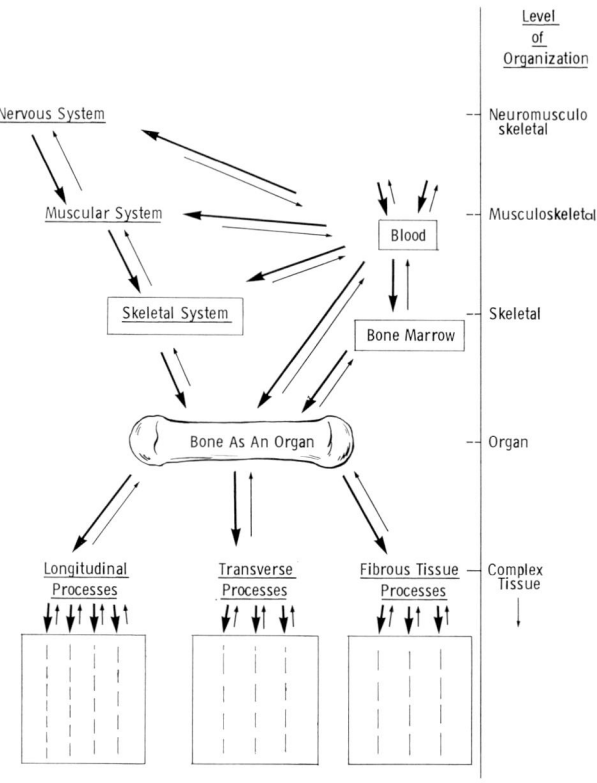

Figure 10.02. Systems Atlas for the Neuromotoskeletal System: On the far right you will find recognizable levels of organization, given names, some of which have appeared previously in this book. At the upper left, the nervous system exerts direct control over the properties and behavior of the musculature (that represents the meaning of the heavy arrows in this series of figures); the interactions of these two systems (now a two-link chain) then affect the properties and behavior of the skeletal system, and that three-link chain then directly affects the behavior and properties of individual bones as organs. The lighter arrows represent feedback, or the fact that reverse effects also occur; in fact, all negative feedback systems require a minimum of two reciprocal routes of informational flow. Three subsystems directly and solely determine the properties of a bone as an organ: the longitudinally acting, transversely acting, and fibrogenetically based properties. The next three figures in this series dissect each more fully. While the previous text has said little of the blood and bone marrow, it was not because they are unimportant, it was because my qualifications to speak on

them cannot match those concerning matters we have discussed. Because of their very real importance you will find them appropriately located on the diagram. The open-ended arrows around the blood signify that it interacts with many other systems too. This diagram covers five levels of organization.

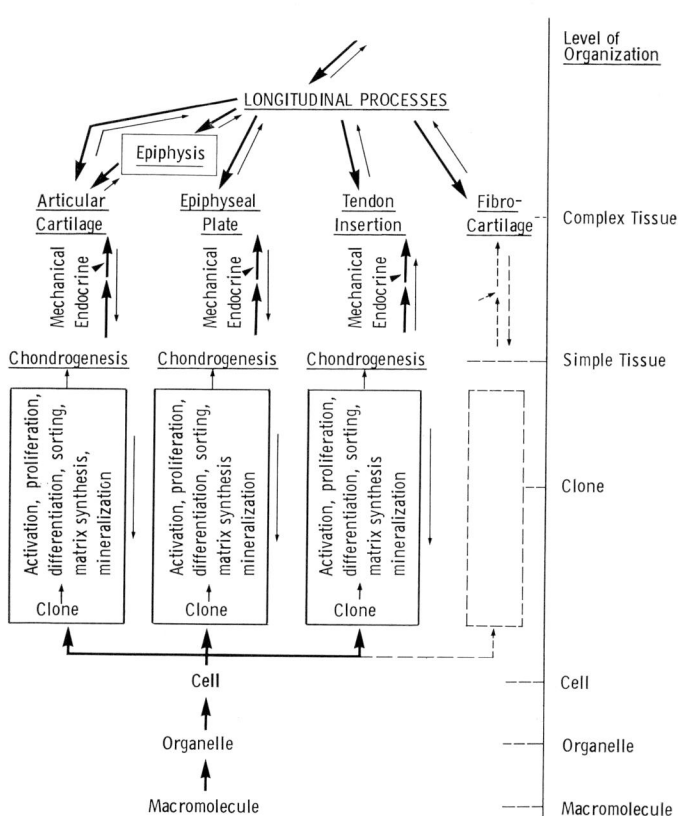

Figure 10.03. This figure expands on the longitudinal processes shown at the complex tissue level in the preceding figure. It identifies but does not dissect in detail two such tissues: epiphyses (which also serve to illustrate the essential properties of apophyses) and fibrocartilage. It does dissect the other three shown and adds five more lower levels of organization to the neuromotoskeletal system below the complex tissue level. The information becomes scanty at and below the clonal level in these figures because of a lack of relevant data; it has not yet occurred to many people that much future progress depends upon getting it.

spongiosa, epiphysis and/or apophysis). As to functions, it establishes in sum the bone's length, its articular architecture, and its content of spongy bone. Earlier chapters described these basic functions, even if briefly so. In the functional sense, the term "compacta" here would include its histogenesis during embryonic life, its subsequent growth and modeling and lifelong turnover or remodeling, and its mechanical functions. We will ignore its blood-bone exchange and marrow interaction functions here. (The last chapters in Volume III will deal with some of their aspects.) The modeling activity sculpts or shapes all of the bone's noncartilaginous surfaces during growth, determining thereby its mass,

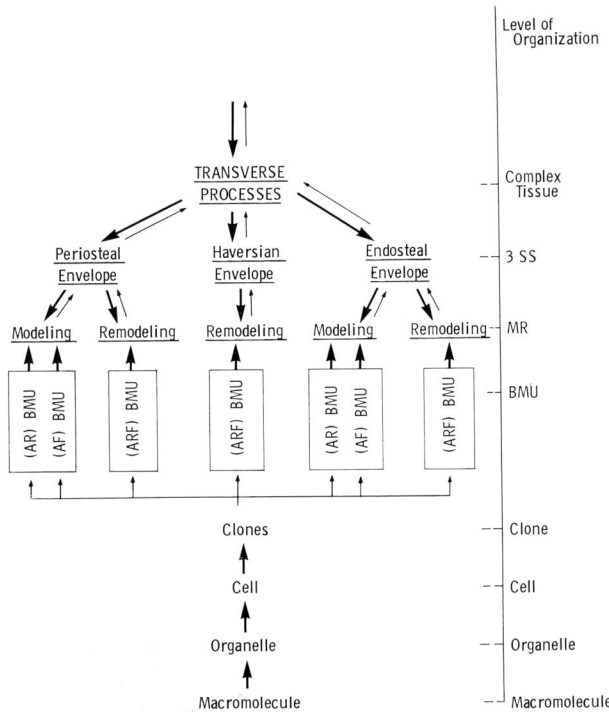

Figure 10.04. Here we dissect the group of transversely acting processes found towards the bottom of Figure 10.02, adding seven new levels of organization below the complex tissue level and including macromolecular properties. Volumes III and IV of this series will go into them in much greater detail. The bulk of this chapter deals with this material.

size, geometry, and mechanical strength properties. The remodeling activity acts to turn over or renew the bony tissue throughout life, constantly replacing old with new and thereby maintaining a material with optimal mechanical, blood-bone exchange, and repair potential.

In this scheme, all of the above represent both behavior and

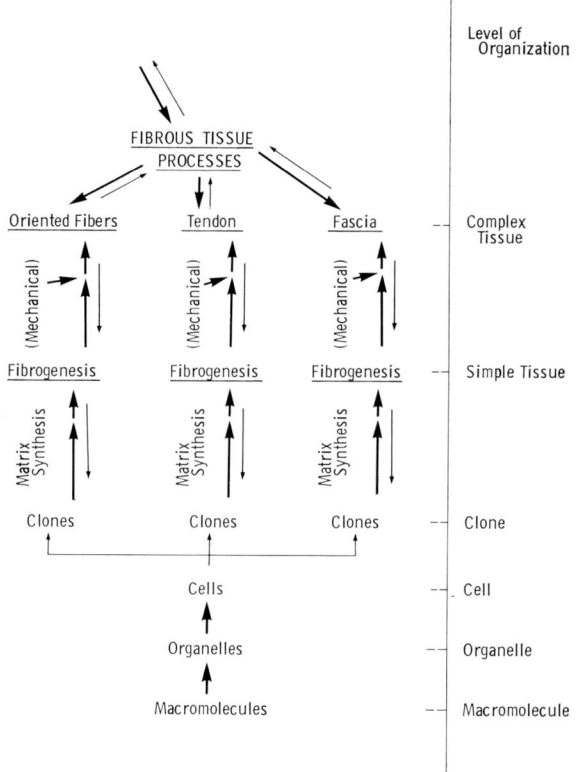

Figure 10.05. This diagram dissects the fibrogenetically based category of complex tissue activities that appears in the box at the bottom right in Figure 10.02, and it adds five levels below the complex tissue level in that figure. The "mechanical" found in parentheses signifies that biomechanical factors arising externally to the fibroblasts that make the collagen affect and in large part determine the overall architecture of the fibrous tissue that develops. The oriented fibril group would include the investing fascia of capillaries, nerves, renal parenchyma, and liver as examples. The other two are self-explanatory.

212   The Physiology of Cartilaginous, Fibrous, and Bony Tissue

functions supplied by only three horizontal categories of activities, all lying at the same complex tissue-level of organization.

At this juncture we encounter three downward-branching dendritic pathways in the organizational map. One stems downwards into the ENOS activities, the other into those of the compacta, the third into fibrogenetic processes. We will take the middle path henceforth and ignore the others.

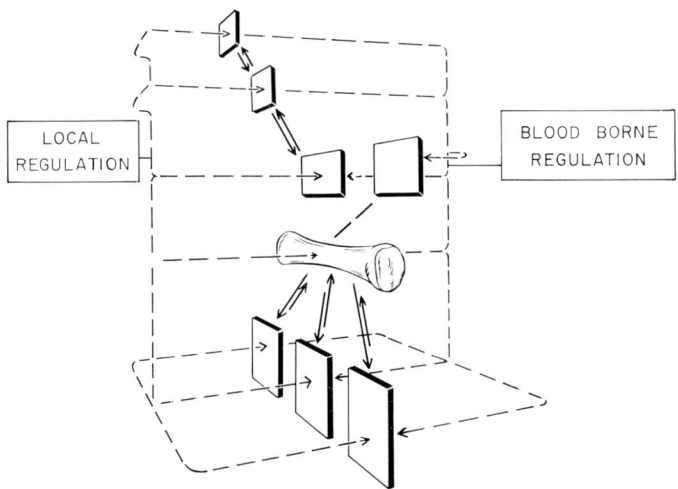

Figure 10.06. This consists of Figure 10.02, now turned sideways to view another "dimension" of the system—that which relates its behavior to the *geographic direct sources* of the factors that regulate that behavior. Three broad categories of such factors exist: (a) those carried to the system by the blood (right), (b) those that arise in the local environment of the tissues and cells (left), and (c) those inherent in the tissue systems and their cells by virtue of their genetically encoded information, which determines their *response characteristics*. These factors act and *interact* at all levels of vertical organization, and the response characteristics (or rules of behavior such as previously described for cartilage and fibrous tissue) of the same cells but at different levels of organization can vary in a manner not predictable from the response characteristics of isolated, individual cells. By turning this figure appropriately, yet another "dimension" of the system can be brought into plain view, that shown in Figure 1.04.

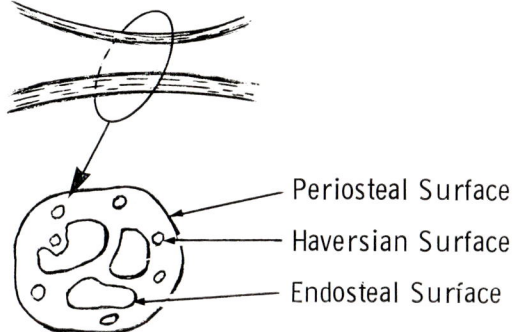

Figure 10.07. Concerning the midshaft region of the bone in the preceding figure, three of its anatomically separable kinds of surfaces also exhibit behavioral and functional properties which justify recognizing each of them as a functionally unique entity. Thus, while all three can (and do) do certain things in unison, under known real circumstances each also does things which the others do not. These surfaces represent the periosteal, haversian, and endosteal *envelopes,* an apt term because each surface does encompass a measureable and characteristic volume of space, one determined by the balance between all previous resorption and formation of bone occurring on that surface.

Triple Surface Level

At this next lower level, we deal only with the compacta, and only as we find it in postnatal life. Here, as Figure 10.04 reveals, three behaviorally independent bone surfaces cooperate in a kind of concert to establish—directly, solely, and via transversely acting accumulations and/or losses of bone—the transverse architectural properties and part of the longitudinal curvatures of a bone during growth and thus, too, the locations in tissue space of the diaphyses relative both to the bone ends and to the musculature which acts on them.

Modeling-Remodeling Level (MR)

The above three surfaces or envelopes undergo simple tissue turnover (i.e. remodeling) throughout life, but the modeling activity only (we believe at present) during growth. Figure 10.08

214 *The Physiology of Cartilaginous, Fibrous, and Bony Tissue*

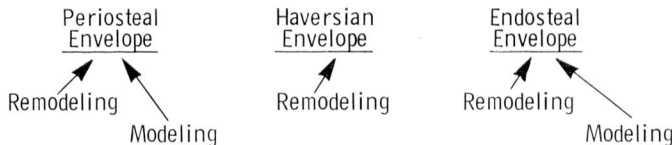

Figure 10.08. Another important item of information abstracted from Figure 10.02 because of its functional and disease-oriented meaning and importance. While remodeling or turnover activity occurs throughout life on all three envelopes, histologically identifiable modeling activity occurs only on the periosteal and endosteal envelopes.

isolates this information from the complex details shown in Figure 10.02.

Thus, the periosteal and marrow cavity walls of children display both modeling and turnover, but after skeletal maturity modeling ceases (for practical purposes at least) and only remodeling remains. The haversian envelope, however, reveals no modeling activity at any age, one of the behavioral properties that set it aside from the other two, as abstracted from Figure 10.04 and shown in Figure 10.08. Let us then ignore the dendrite that leads down to modeling, henceforth, and consider further only the lower organizational details of remodeling.

Remodeling activity turns over the bony tissue in the skeleton several complete times during a normal lifespan, thereby replacing old and possibly worn-out portions of the skeleton with new, to maintain optimum functional competence. It produces little and probably only very slow (i.e. over decades of time) changes in the total, net amounts of bone in various parts of the skeleton, unlike modeling, which can produce rapid (i.e. over months) and large changes. Figure 10.09 diagrams the levels of organization lying below the remodeling level.

The BMU Level

A BMU signifies a complex histological and functional multicellular unit. Analogous to the nephron in the kidney, and signifying *B*asic *M*ulticellular *U*nit, it supplies "packets" or action quanta of the bone removal and bone-building activities involved

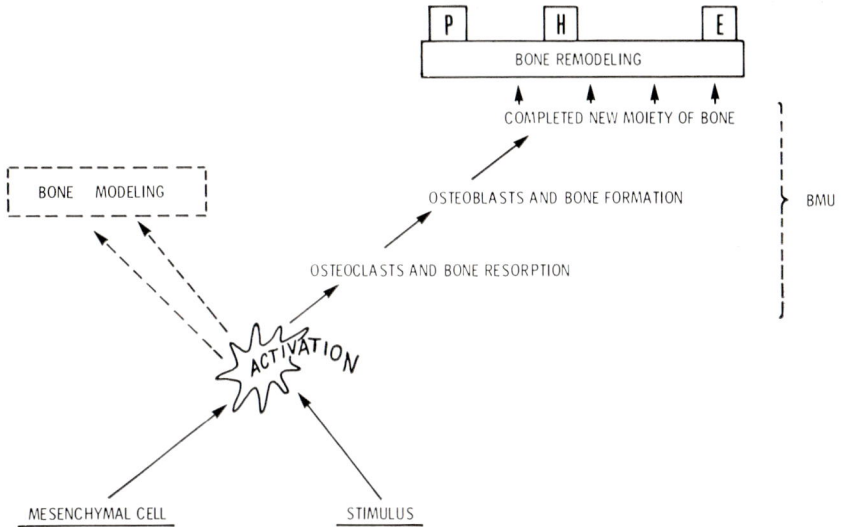

Figure 10.09. This figure isolates additional information, this time from Figure 10.04. Specifically, remodeling has underlying and more elementary determinants which, via specific and identifiable cause-effect chains, derive ultimately from a large number of cells and thence macromolecules. The typical functional unit or module at any given level represents an association of two or more kinds of more elementary units. Thus, a gland would be the sum of its acini, and its acini the sum of its individual cells.

in adult bone physiology and in bone turnover. The summed-up contributions of thousands of BMU annually create skeletal-level bone remodeling. The third volume in this series will have a lot to say about BMU and their behavioral properties. In any realistic understanding of bone physiology they assume the same role as nephrons do in understanding renal physiology.

At the Clonal Level

The cellular proliferative, differentiative, and associative events which provide the cells in a BMU and which determine its inherent behavioral properties *and its response characteristics to pharmacologic, endocrine, and biomechanical factors* represent clonal phenomena, at present nearly totally unstudied insofar as they pertain to bone modeling and remodeling.

216   *The Physiology of Cartilaginous, Fibrous, and Bony Tissue*

At the Cellular and Lower Levels

Here arise the cellular activities whose associations underlie and determine clonal level properties; they arise in turn from *organelle level* activities, which in their turn derive from *macromolecular level* activities. Figure 10.10 diagrams the terminology involved and the relationships between the activities signified by the terms.

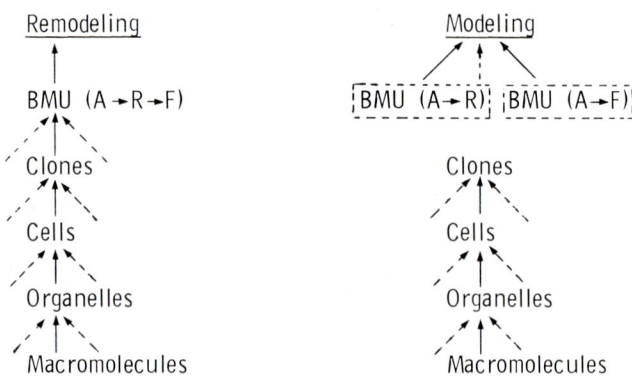

Figure 10.10. This simply shows by means of a diagram the etymological and morphological relations between some of the terms that appear in this book, as an aid to understanding them. Such a diagram has value because some of the terms and the activities they stand for do not yet appear in standard texts or medical dictionaries, although the identity of the activities and relationships they signify no longer form subjects of legitimate controversy; the evidence for their existence is too unequivocal and obvious.

Let us now consider two examples of how this particular trajectory of cause-effect within the skeletal systems atlas expedited research into skeletal physiological and pathophysiological problems. These will consist of postmenopausal osteoporosis and the mechanism via which growth hormone accelerates bone formation at the organ and higher levels of the neuromusculoskeletal system.

Postmenopausal Osteoporosis

In its senile (SO) and postmenopausal (PMO) forms, osteoporosis afflicts a significant fraction of our elder citizens, particularly the women, whose skeletons during adult life come to contain too little bone tissue which, furthermore, has become thin and fragile. As the average age of our population gradually increases, this disease poses an increasingly pressing problem, and it has attracted a great deal of attention from investigators as well as in the medical and lay presses.

The absolute loss of bone found in the skeletons of these patients implies an imbalance, such that bone resorption exists in relative excess over formation (Johnson[53]). Strategically speaking, one might search for a cure for this excess in two extreme ways: By trying various treatments on a random basis as I defined "random" in the previous chapter (which, although the approach commonly used in the 20 years leading up to and including this time of writing, nevertheless reduces nearly to zero the probability of therapeutic or systems control capability success), or by using some systematized strategy such as the one described here. To abstract much effort and detail,* a systems-analytical approach to this disease in our Orthopaedic Research Laboratory greatly sharpened and fundamentally redirected the focus of our own attention, and its results have now begun to receive serious attention outside of Detroit. Consider the following facts and reasoning, referring back to Figure 10.02 as needed. The theme of the analysis for the moment will constitute *direct mechanical causality* as we trace the cause-effect chain in this disease downwards, layer by layer, as follows:

1. We can begin by dispensing with the top two levels of organization in the neuromotoskeletal system in that figure, for PMO appears as a disease of bone, such that it becomes subject to fracture under normal (and normally patterned) muscular contractile forces. In one move that single fact takes us down to the skeleton.

---

*The initial work often went on false paths because the concepts of research strategy outlined here were evolving simultaneously and equally erratically.

2. Study of PMO skeletons by divers means shows an absolute loss of bony tissue, but one which reaches its greatest extent in the axial as opposed to the appendicular skeleton.

Further observations indicate that that loss of bone occurred during adult life. Here two simple facts become relevant: Both endochondral ossification and modeling activity cease at about age 18 years, but remodeling activity continues throughout life. Then, if postmenopausal osteoporosis develops during adult life, our systems atlas in Figure 10.02 immediately points to the remodeling activities as the probable source of the causative abnormality. Note that this comparison of normal to abnormal has also, and at one additional move, eliminated 66 per cent of the information at the skeletal level in that figure as probably trivial to the present quest.

4. At the next layer, the 3ss or triple surface system, simple comparison of bone envelope sizes in normal skeletons with the skeletons of women with postmenopausal osteoporosis show quite clearly that bone loss characterizing the latter occurs primarily (although not exclusively) on cortical-endosteal and trabecular bone surfaces, without abnormal bone gain or loss on the other two surfaces (Wu et al[106]). In other words, the bone loss developed *only on those surfaces in physical contact with the marrow tissues;* a wide variety of studies and many different investigators concur in this.

Thus, in three simple moves we have now classified and specified eight-ninths of all potential skeletal-level possibilities as irrelevant to this quest, in the process also locating where in the systems atlas the remaining one-ninth of the information relevant to a systems controls capability goal does (or at least should) exist. The above simple and widely known facts (but, before we identified their significance by the means now undergoing review, little discussed) then initiated two separate lines of new work in our laboratory: (a) a histological search for the mechanically most direct cellular cause of the cortical-endosteal bone loss, and (b) a deductive analysis of some of the general features of its ultimate regulatory cause(s). The following is relative to the former (a):

5. *The BMU Level:* With respect to direct mechanical cause and about 20 years ago, osteoblasts and osteoclasts were assumed to comprise two functionally independent collections of cells (see Rasmussen and Tenehouse[74]), a concept I dub the "independence assumption." In principle, that assumption implies that some kinds of pharmacologic "cocktails" exist which would increase only the output of osteoblasts or decrease only the output of osteoclasts, and that they would do that throughout the skeleton generally, meaning on all three of its surfaces or envelopes. But, and while such a cocktail may indeed someday prove to exist (although not properly conveyed in the oversimplified manner just employed), the fact that the bone loss characterizing PMO occurs only on the endosteal envelope makes it quite clear that such a systemic effect on all bone cells cannot cause postmenopausal osteoporosis nor would invoking its antithesis provide an ideal cure. Further on that line, we have shown in the past that in fact a consistent and close operational association usually exists between osteoclasts and osteoblasts as they participate in adult bone remodeling. One finds them "tethered" in the earlier mentioned BMU, as "packets" of bone-formative activity; this sequence occurs on a definite time scale and follows a definite spatial orientation in the bone. In other words, while an acceptable first approximation try, the independence assumption proved false as it applies to bone remodeling.

If, in the direct sense, remodeling BMU on the endosteal envelope causes PMO, one next asks, How? To find out, we extrapolated five theoretically possible causal endosteal BMU mechanisms to their necessary morphological effects on bone, and by comparing normal bones to those of patients with PMO, searched for evidence of any of them in the tissues of the latter. One of them, representing augmented bone removal per typical endosteal BMU, did then emerge as the most likely direct cause of the disease (Wu *et al*[102]). Thus, using the systems atlas described earlier, and by means of one additional strategic move, we have picked out 1/6 x 1/9 or 1/54th part of the total information in the intact skeletal system which seems to contain the therapeutically oriented answers most of us seek relative to PMO.

Note that in theory the magnitude of this bone loss depends directly on only two independent variables in the BMU system: The relative and absolute magnitudes of the excess of resorption over formation per BMU and the total number of BMU created over a period of time on the entire endosteal bone surface (of which more shortly)—in homelier terms: Either bigger BMU "bites" out of the marrow cavity walls, or many more than the normal number of bites, or some of both. Our present work in this area focuses on these two possibilities but does not yet allow further specification of the causal defect(s) at lower levels of organization in this system (which comprise the clonal and cellular levels).

> *Nota bene:* Here I cannot and do not claim any greater intelligence than my colleagues around the world who also concern themselves with PMO, and certainly I have not had better financial backing than many of them enjoyed and still enjoy (Our typical grant funds averaged $20,000 per annum over the 1958-67 period that the A. M. division of N. I. H. supported our work). The above strategy which I now try to give away gratis put our intellectual faculties to efficient and effective use *by minimizing the number of false paths our work followed.* Thereby we accomplished as much if not more in those nine years than any competitors in this area did in any number of years. Paraphrased, a mediocre tool under proper guidance can do far better cabinet work than the most expensive tool available in misguided hands.

6. *Geographic Locus of the Direct Cause:* With respect to the site of action of its systemic cause, recognition that PMO constituted a bone surface-specific disease completely upended all of our previous thinking. Like the majority of other scientists interested in PMO, I originally simply assumed that the systemic, blood-borne abnormality which probably caused it *did so by acting directly on bone cells.* This would imply equal behavioral effects on these cells wherever they exist, and I call that the "singularity assumption." It means as an example that one assumes that all of the body's osteoblasts comprise a single functional group of cells, in the sense that everywhere in the anatomical sense they respond similarly to any change in a circulating regulatory agent. Obviously, some truth and logic exist in such a view, the very factors which up to now have prevented

our profession from facing and dealing with the alternative possibility that in some real circumstances truth and logic might not apply. Such a concept naturally might lead one to study the actions of regulatory agents (suspected as causally involved) on living bone cells in highly sophisticated *in vitro* systems. Much very expensive research expertise has attempted by means of such systems to define the actions on osteoclasts and osteoblasts of fluoride, parathormone, calcium, vitamin D, thyrocalcitonin, acid-base equilibrium, sex hormones, adrenal corticosteroids, phosphonates, and the like.

While we certainly need such information as it applies to skeletal physiology generally, as far as PMO goes, such an approach has taken us up a dead-end street. In support thereof, witness: The surface-specific nature of the bone loss in osteoporosis unequivocally points to the presence of some *anatomically localized mediating regulatory factor*, furthermore one confined to the bone marrow cavity. Thus, in PMO the singularity assumption does not apply.

We have now located $1/2 \times 1/54 =$ that 1/108th part of the skeletal system which holds the answers to this particular search: The secret lies in some interaction occurring between the marrow cavity and endosteal bone cells.

Now consider an interesting question which answers itself: If you had a way of increasing by a factor of 108x the probability that your own research would prove directly relevant to your research goal, would you then ignore it? Of course not.

At this time, the assembled evidence relative to PMO strongly points to something associated with hematopoietic activity in the bone marrow as the mediating factor referred to in the preceding paragraph. That factor constitutes the *direct* target of any systemic cause(s) of osteoporosis; the then-altered marrow somehow influences the behavior of the bone cells near it, causing each endosteal BMU to remove an excessive amount of cortical-endosteal or trabecular bone.

7. Finally, other comparisons of bone dynamics in PMO with normal have revealed additional features typical of the PMO state. They consist of modestly decreased bone turnover gener-

ally, and a markedly slowed rate of BMU-based production of new packets of bone. The latter provides an acceptable hypothetical explanation for spontaneous fractures in PMO, for it retards the repair of mechanical microdamage to the bone and so could allow the latter to progress faster than the remodeling process can repair it. In time the accumulation of microdamage caused by such a relationship could well lead to a gross fracture under normal mechanical loads.

8. Thus, a really quite simple *downwards systems analysis* pointed to the bone marrow tissue as the direct target of the systemic cause(s) of PMO. This would explain (I hasten to point out, not the same thing as *does* explain) why so little progress has been made in the past in terms of curing the actual disease by expending millions of dollars, man hours, and experimental animals in the effort; the *strategy* underlying most of these efforts practically doomed them at their inceptions, for they all assumed the independence and singularity properties represented exclusive reality. We know now, and beyond any reasonable doubt, that they contain serious deficiencies (and to any critics who might observe that I have not cured PMO yet either, I concede the point).

CONTROL OF THE BONE FORMATION RATE

If a behavioral prediction generated by a new hypothesis violates common belief as well as what seems to represent common sense, it usually evokes incredulity. If observation subsequently verifies such a prediction, its underlying theory then receives more serious consideration. The following paragraphs deal with exactly such a situation, one that popped up in the form of the mode of action of growth hormone on skeletal physiology. Keep in mind during the following paragraphs that physiologists who have not caught up to date on recent bone studies still widely believe that growth hormone (STH) acts directly upon osteoblasts to increase the rate and total quantity of bone they produce individually. This has even been proposed (and possibly in that case with some justice) to explain the greater overall bone-forming activity in children compared to that in adults.

Define *cell-level bone formation* as the bone made per osteoblast in unit time (it occurs at the third-from-the-bottom level in Fig. 10.04); define *tissue-level formation* as cell-level formation times the number of osteoblasts in a unit amount of bone tissue, such as in a gram or milliliter (that occurs at the complex tissue level and at all higher levels in Fig. 10.02). Then a conventional view would state that activity at the latter level follows directly and proportionally that at the former. This view sneaks in under its coat-tails the major corollary assumption that, as one ascends from the cellular to the tissue level of skeletal organization, no new variables enter the system which could independently affect tissue-level bone formation. That view conflicts seriously with the system's atlas sketched briefly already (and in a way described in detail in the next volume), for between the cell and the organ's complex tissue level that atlas identifies at least four potential such variables (see Fig. 10.04). We shall now examine this assumption.

Morphologic and tritiated thymidine studies summarized by Young,[104] Johnson[53] and myself (reference 36) reveal that new osteoblasts usually arise from mesenchymal cells *de novo*, in discrete batches of 10^3 to 10^5 cells, and in the microscopic bony locale where they will function. In a human remodeling BMU, such a batch of osteoblasts makes a new microscopic moiety of bone in a period of about three months and it then disappears (Frost[36]). Since at least 95 per cent of the body's normal bone turnover represents the additive contributions of many discrete BMU, each containing its own batch of osteoblasts, bone formation then should occur in discrete "packets" (i.e. BMU); various studies directed specifically to that matter have verified that point.[98, 102]

As to the size of these "packets," several investigators report independently the peculiar behavioral property that, regardless of how quickly or slowly the osteoblasts made it, the average amount of new bone contained in completed ones varied relatively little with age and disease ($\pm 20\%$) and in different bones ($\pm 40\%$); see for example Currey,[18, 19] Landeros and Frost,[56] and Arnold and Bartley.[4] Yet our own tetracycline-labeling studies show that,

224 The Physiology of Cartilaginous, Fibrous, and Bony Tissue

in real life, tissue-level bone formation rates can range over approximately four magnitudes, or 10,000/1.[98]

If bone formation occurs in BMU packets as stated earlier, and if *on the average* each contributes a constant amount of new bone (actually this represents a Markovian type of constancy), then when a steady state exists with respect to packet initiations and completions, bone formation in the whole skeleton should come to depend primarily *and only* on their population dynamics. It forms an elementary theoretical problem (see *Mathematical Elements of Lamellar Bone Remodeling*, Springfield, Thomas, 1964) to show that the following two properties should characterize the output behavior of any such system over long spans of time:

1. The frequency of packet creations in a unit amount of tissue should determine the average, steady-state level of bone forming activity in that unit of tissue.

2. The average tissue-level activity could proceed independently of cellular level activity; that is, one could proceed supernormally and the other subnormally, or the converse, or in any other combination.

Figure 10.11 summarizes the results of work which verified these somewhat novel predictions for the case of haversian bone remodeling in man (Villanueva and Frost[98]).

In effect, this figure says that whatever changes growth hormone *(and all other regulatory factors)* may exert on the steady state tissue-level bone formation rate, it does so by the simple expedient of changing the *numbers* of new packets of bone *initiated* in unit time, and it does so completely independently of any additional changes it might also cause in how quickly (or slowly) the individual osteoblasts in each packet subsequently produce their own little moiety of bone. While that may prove hard to understand, it constitutes a fact—and an example of the different concepts mentioned in the last paragraph in the preface. Thus, the important physiological effect of growth hormone in this system does not appear in individual osteoblasts; *the important action of the hormone affects their progenitor cells.*

No wonder that talented and sophisticated biochemical efforts to demonstrate enhanced protein synthesis per cell in *in vitro*

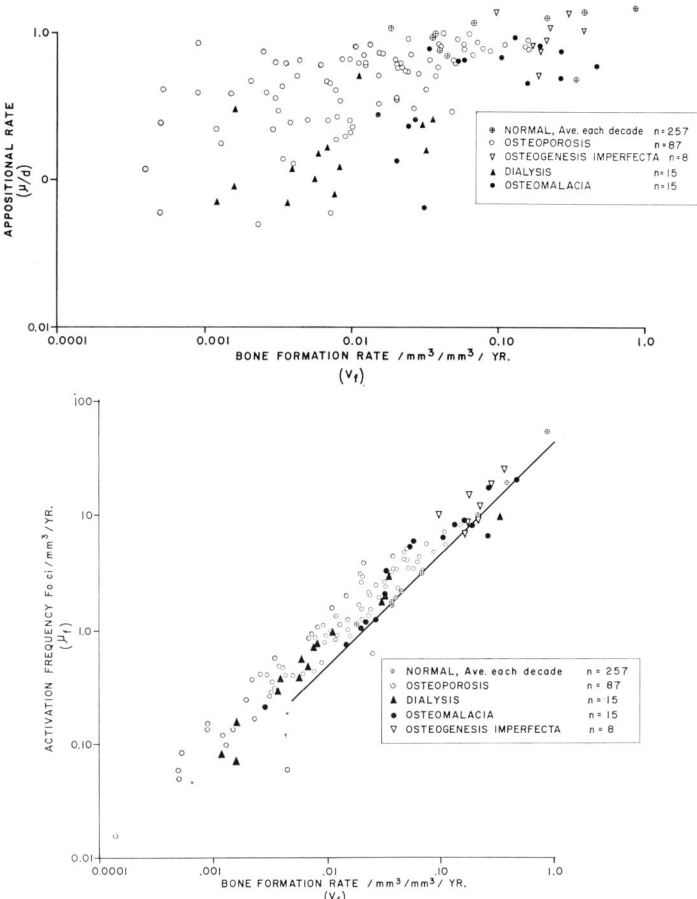

Figure 10.11. Both of these graphs plot data from the same group of tetracycline-labeled rib biopsies taken from 382 humans, some medically and skeletally healthy, and some with a variety of diseases identified by the inscriptions. On both graphs, both axes are logarithmic; on both, the horizontal axis plots for each patient his *tissue level* bone formation rate. *Top:* For each person, the vertical axis plots a reliable index of cellular-level bone formation against his tissue-level bone formation. Clearly one could not use a known value on one axis to make a usefully accurate prediction of the value on the other. *Bottom:* Now we plot on the vertical axis the number of new packets initiated or "born" in unit time against tissue level bone formation. Clearly, one can serve to predict the other with useful accuracy.

226   The Physiology of Cartilaginous, Fibrous, and Bony Tissue

In other words, cell population dynamics, not biochemical factors in the classical sense, account for changes in skeletal bony anabolic and catabolic activity in health and in disease. (Reprinted by permission, A. R. Villanueva and H. M. Frost, *J Dent Res* 49:836, 1970.)

systems by treatment with STH failed to do so, although a clear enhancement of protein synthesis occurs *per intact animal*. The initial strategy underlying such studies doomed them to fail to explain these bodily effects of STH from the very beginning. Biochemists have shown some reluctance to accept such concepts when they come from mere morphologists or dunderheaded clinicians dabbling in morphology, but biological science is a chain, and when one's career hangs suspended on such he ignores links other than his special very own at his own peril.

Concluding Remarks

The above two examples illustrate, admittedly briefly and partially, what might follow applying a more efficient systems-analytical strategy to the study of a strategically poorly developed biological system, the skeleton. We must consider that the skeleton does still remain a very poorly developed system, until such time as we have acquired the ability to cure quite a few more of its ailments and creaks than the relatively few we now can cure, and until such time as we can extend all of the dendrites of Figure 10.02 down to their real macromolecular-level bases.

QUESTIONS

1. An investigator proposes that a specific enzyme defect in hyaline cartilage cells causes the deformities of Morquio's disease. What anatomical sites might one biopsy to obtain reasonable assurance that he will obtain tissue which would demonstrate such a defect, were the proposal correct?
2. A student in anatomy proposes to define in rats the differences in chemical composition that characterize bones formed in the ontogenic sense in membrane, and bones formed in cartilage. Evaluate.

Application of Strategy

3. A variety of studies reveals that increased protein synthesis and catabolism (i.e. turnover) arise at the body and organ levels in thyrotoxicosis. Evaluate the research proposal to explain that idea in a cell-culture system as an acceleratory effect of T_4 on protein synthetic intracellular pathways; for STH; for testosterone.

4. In screening synthetic adrenal-cortical steroid compounds for any adverse osteoporosis-producing effect, a drug company takes as an index of the "bone effect" measurements of the thickness of the proximal tibial epiphyseal plates in treated young rats. Evaluate.

5. You just examined a 48-year-old male patient applying for permanent, total disability as the consequence of a work-related injury to his lower back three years previously. Since that injury he has only worked five months at his job of punch-press operator, he has had two laminectomies (L-4-5) and a spinal fusion (solid on x-rays taken during bending), and has not worked at all during the previous one year, all because of disabling low back pain with radiation down the left lower extremity.

His physical findings include 1.5 cm atrophy left calf, weak left extensor hallucis longus, no detectable differences in comparison x-rays of both feet, heavy and equal wear of his right and left shoes, straight leg-raising positive for severe back pain on the left at only 10,° a painful callosity under the second metatarsal head on the left, and a marked limp of the pain-protective (i.e. shortened stance phase) type on the left lower while walking.

What kind of disability does this man almost certainly exhibit? Physical or psychogenic? Outline your reasoning.

Bibliography

1. Aegerter, E. E., and Kirkpatrick, J. A.: *Orthopaedic Diseases*, 2nd ed. Philadelphia, W. B. Saunders, 1962.
2. Amprino, R., and Marotti, G.: A topographic quantitative study of bone formation and reconstruction. In E. J. J. Blackwood (Ed): *Bone and Tooth Symposium*. New York, Macmillan, 1964, pp. 21-33.
3. Apter, M. J., and Wolpert, L.: Cybernetics and development. I: Information theory, *J Theor Biol 8*:244-257, 1965.
4. Arnold, J. S., Bartley, M. H., Tont, S. A., and Jenkins, D. P.: Skeletal changes in aging and disease. *Clin Orthop 49*:17-38, 1966.
5. Arnold, J. S.: Focal excessive endosteal resorption in aging and senile osteoporosis. In U. S. Barzel (Ed): *Osteoporosis*. New York, Grune and Stratton, 1970, pp. 80-113.
6. Arnold, J. S.: Personal communication.
7. Arnstein, A. R., and Frame, B.: Primary hypophosphatemic rickets and osteomalacia: A review. *Clin Orthop 49*:109-118, 1966.
8. Ashby, W. R.: *An Introduction to Cybernetics*. New York, John Wiley and Sons, 1963.
9. Baker, S. L., Dent, C. E., Friedman, M., and Watson, L.: Fibrogenesis imperfecta ossium. *J Bone Joint Surg 48B*:804-825, 1966.
10. Bassett, C. A. L.: Biological significance of piezoelectricity. *Calcif Tissue Res 1*:252-272, 1968.
11. Becker, R. O.: The bioelectric field pattern in the salamander and its simulation by an electronic analog. *I.R.E. Trans Med Electron 7*:202-207, 1960.
12. Becker, R. O., Bassett, C. A. L., and Bachman, C. H.: Bioelectrical factors controlling bone structure. In *Bone Biodynamics*. Boston, Little, Brown, 1964, pp. 209-232.
13. Belanger, L. F., Robichon, J., Migicovsky, B. B., Copp, D. H., and Vincent, J.: Resorption without osteoclasts (osteolysis). In R. F. Sognnaes, (Ed): *Mechanics of Hard Tissue Destruction*. Washington, D. C., A. A. A. S., 1963, pp. 531-556.
14. Berliner, D. L., Bartley, M. H., Kenner, G. H., and Jee, W. S. S.: Activity of antiinflammatory steroids upon fibroblasts and bones. *Br J Dermatol 82*:53-61, 1970.
15. Collins, E. J., and Baker, V. F.: Growth hormone and radiosulfate incorporation: A new assay method for growth hormone. *Metabolism 9*:556-560, 1960.

16. Coutelier, L.: Recherches sur la guèrison des fractures. Brussels, *Ed Arscia S. A.*, 1969.
17. Currey, J. D.: Stress concentrations in bone. *Q J Microscop Sci 10:* 111-333, 1962.
18. Currey, J. D.: Three analogies to explain the mechanical properties of bone. *Biorheology 2:*1-10, 1964.
19. Currey, J. D.: The adaptations of bones to stress. *J Theor Biol 20:*91-106, 1968.
20. DeBroyn, P. D. H., Breen, P. C., and Thomas, T. B.: The microcirculation of the bone marrow. *Anat Rec 168:*55-68, 1970.
21. Duncan, H.: Paget's disease of bone (ostetic deformans). In Tice: *Practice of Medicine.* Baltimore, Harper & Row, 1969, ch. 5, p. 54.
22. Eisenberg, E.: Effect of androgens, estrogens and corticoids on strontium kinetics in man. *J Clin Endocrinol Metab 26:*566-572, 1966.
23. Enlow, D. H.: Functions of the haversian system. *Am J Anat 110:*269-306, 1962.
24. Enlow, D. H.: *Principles of Bone Remodeling.* Springfield, Thomas, 1963.
25. Enlow, D. H.: Wolff's law and the factor of architectonic circumstance. *Am J Orthod 54:*803-822, 1968.
26. Enlow, D. H., and Brown, S. O.: A comparative histological study of fossil and recent bone tissues. *Texas J Sci 10:*187-230, 1958.
27. Epker, B. N.: Studies on bone turnover and balance in the rabbit. I: Effects of hydrocortisone. *Clin Orthop 72:*315-326, 1970.
28. Feinstein, A. R.: What kind of basic science for clinical medicine? *N Engl J Med 283:*847-852, 1970.
29. Firschein, H. E.: Collagen and mineral dynamics in bone. *Clin Orthop 66:*212-225, 1969.
30. Frame, B., and Nixon, R. K.: Bone marrow factors in osteoporosis. In U. S. Barzel (Ed): *Osteoporosis.* New York, Grune and Stratton, 1970, pp. 238-250.
31. Frame, B.: Personal communication.
32. Frost, H. M.: Osteoporosis: A hard look. *J Am Gerontol Soc 8:*568-571, 1960.
33. Frost, H. M.: *Laws of Bone Structure.* Springfield, Thomas, 1964.
34. Frost, H. M.: *Bone Dynamics in Osteoporosis and Osteomalacia.* Springfield, Thomas, 1966.
35. Frost, H. M.: *Introduction to Biomechanics.* Springfield, Thomas, 1966.
36. Frost, H. M.: Tetracycline based analysis of bone remodeling. *Calcified Tissue Res 3:*211-237, 1969.
37. Frost, H. M., and Arnold, J. S.: The osteocyte as a bone pump. *Clin Orthop. 78:*47-55, 1971.
38. Garn, S. M.: *The Earlier Gain and the Later Loss of Cortical Bone.* Springfield, Thomas, 1970.

39. Gendreau, C. L.: Thesis: *Osteogenesis of the Capital Femoral Epiphysis of the Dog.* University of Guelph, Ontario, 1970, pp. 1-120.
40. Gong, J. K., Arnold, J. S., and Cohn, S. T.: Composition of trabecular and cortical bone. *Anat Rec* 149:325-322, 1964.
41. Goss, R. J.: Hypertrophy vs. hyperplasia. *Science* 153:1615-1620, 1966.
42. Gram, R. B., Fleming, J. L., Frame, B., and Fine, G.: Metaphyseal chondrodysplasia of Jansen. *J Bone Joint Surg* 41A:951-959, 1959.
43. Haas, H. G., Muller, J., and Shenk, R. K.: Osteomalacia: Metabolic and quantitative histologic studies. *Clin Orthop* 53:213-222, 1967.
44. Hall, B. K.: Histogenesis and morphogenesis of bone. *Clin Orthop* 74: 249-268, 1971.
45. Hancox, N. M.: The osteoclast. *Biol Rev* 24:448-471, 1949.
46. Harris, W. H., and Heaney, R. P.: Skeletal renewal and metabolic bone disease. *N Engl J Med* 280:303-311, 1969.
47. Heaney, R. P.: Interpretation of calcium kinetic data. In *Dynamic Studies of Metabolic Bone Disease.* Philadelphia, F. A. Davis, 1964, pp. 11-23.
48. Hohl, J.: Personal communication.
49. Jacob, F., and Monod, J.: Genetic regulatory mechanisms in the synthesis of proteins. *J Mol Biol* 3:318-356, 1961.
50. Jaffe, H. L.: *Tumors and Tumorous Conditions of Bones and Joints.* Philadelphia, Lea and Febiger, 1958.
51. Jee, W. S. S., Blackwood, E. L., Dockum, N. L., Haslam, R. K., and Kincl, F. A.: Bioassay of responses of growing bones to cortisol. *Clin Orthop* 49:39-63, 1966.
52. Jee, W. S. S.: Personal communication.
53. Johnson, L. C.: Morphologic analysis in pathology: The kinetics of disease and general biology of bone. In H. M. Frost (Ed): *Bone Biodynamics.* Boston, Little, Brown, 1964, pp. 543-654.
54. Klein, L., Vessely, J. C., and Heiple, K. G.: Quantification of ^{3}H collagen loss of rat allografted and isografted tendon. *J Bone Joint Surg* 51A:891-898, 1963.
55. Lacroix, P.: *The Organization of Bones.* London, Churchill, 1951.
56. Landeros, O., and Frost, H. M.: A cell system in which the rate and amount of protein synthesis are separately controlled. *Science* 145: 1323-1324, 1964.
57. Lee, W. R.: A quantitative microscopic study of bone formation in a normal child and in two children suffering with osteogenesis imperfecta. *Calcified Tissues,* Belgium, University of Liège, 1964, pp. 451-463.
58. Luck, J. V.: *Bone and Joint Diseases.* Springfield, Thomas, 1950.
59. Mankin, H. J., and Lippiello, L.: The turnover of adult rabbit articular cartilage. *J Bone Joint Surg* 51:862-874, 1969.

60. Marotti, G.: Quantitative studies on bone reconstruction. *Acta Anat 52:* 291-333, 1963.
61. Marshall, J. H.: The retention of radionuclides in bone. In C. W. Mays, W. S. S. Jee, et al (Eds): *Delayed Effects of Bone-Seeking Radionuclides.* Salt Lake City, University of Utah Press, 1969, pp. 7-27.
62. Marshall, J. H., and Onkelinx, C.: Radial diffusion and power function retention of alkaline earth radioisotopes. *Nature 217:*742-743, 1968.
63. Maximow, A. A., and Bloom, Wm.: *A Text Book of Histology*, 6th ed. Philadelphia, W. B. Saunders, 1955.
64. Mayr, E.: Cause and effect in biology. *Science 134:*1501-1506, 1961.
65. McLean, F. C., and Urist, M. R.: *Bone: An Introduction to the Physiology of Skeletal Tissue*, 2nd ed. Chicago, University of Chicago Press, 1961.
66. McMaster, J. H., and Weinert, C. R., Jr.: Effects of mechanical forces on growing cartilage. *Clin Orthop 72:*308-314, 1970.
67. Meunier, P., Vignon, G., and Vauzelle, J. L.: Methodes histologiques quantitatives en pathologie osseuse. *Rev Lyon Med 28:*133-142, 1969.
68. Meunier, P.: Personal communication.
69. Moffett, B. C., Johnson, L. C., McCabe, J. B., and Askew, H. C.: Articular remodeling of the adult human temporomandibular joint. *Am J Anat 115:*119-142, 1964.
70. Nordin, B. E. D., Young, M. M., Bulosu, L., and Horsman, A.: Osteoporosis reexamined. In U. S. Barzel (Ed): *Osteoporosis.* New York, Grune and Stratton, 1970, pp. 47-67.
71. Polanyi, M.: Life's irreducible structure. *Science 160:*1308-1312, 1968.
72. Putschar, W. G. J.: General pathology of the musculoskeletal system. In *Handbuch der Allgemeinen Pathologie.* Heidelberg, Springer-Verlag, 1960, pp. 364-488.
73. Ramser, J. R., Villaneuva, A. R., Pirok, D., and Frost, H. M.: Tetracycline based measurement of bone dynamics in three women with osteogenesis imperfecta. *Clin Orthop 49:*151-162, 1966.
74. Rasmussen, H., and Tenenhouse, A.: Thyrocalcitonin, osteoporosis and osteolysis. *Am J Med 43:*711-726, 1967.
75. Reiner, J. M.: Enzyme kinetics and tissue dynamics. In *Bone Biodynamics.* Boston, Little, Brown, 1964, pp. 59-70.
76. Rindfleisch, E.: *A Manual of Pathological Histology.* London, New Sydenhaum Society, 1873, Vol. II, pp. 271-272.
77. Robinson, R. N., and Elliott, S. R.: Water content of bone. *J Bone Joint Surg 39A:*167-188, 1957.
78. Romer, A. S.: *Vertebrate Paleontology*, 3rd ed. Chicago, University of Chicago Press, 1966.
79. Rubin, P.: *Dynamic Classification of Bone Dysplasias.* Chicago, Year Book Medical Publishers, 1964.

80. Rutishauser, E., and Majno, G.: Lesion osseuse par surcharge dans le squellette normal et pathologique. *Bull Schweiz Akad Med Wiss* 6:333-342, 1950.
81. Salter, R.: *Textbook of Disorders and Injuries of the Musculoskeletal System.* Baltimore, Williams and Wilkins, 1970.
82. Sedlin, E. D.: Uses of bone as a model system in the study of aging. In *Bone Biodynamics.* Boston, Little, Brown, 1964, pp. 655-668.
83. Shannon, C. E., and Weaver, W.: *The Mathematical Theory of Communication.* Chicago, University of Illinois Press, 1963.
84. Shifrin, L. Z.: Correlation of serum alkaline phosphatase with bone formation rates. *Clin Orthop* 70:212-215, 1970.
85. Shifrin, L. Z.: Giant cell tumor of bone. *Clin Orthop.* 1971. In press.
86. Shock, Charles: Personal communication.
87. Smith, J. W.: The relationship of epiphyseal plates to stress in some bones of the lower limb. *J Anat* 90:58-78, 1970.
88. Stanisavljevic, S.: Personal communication.
89. Stanisavljevic, S.: *Diagnosis and Treatment of Congenital Hip Pathology in the Newborn.* Baltimore, Williams and Wilkins, 1964.
90. Stanisavljevic, S., and Mitchell, C. L.: An anatomical-pathological study of congenital hip dysplasia, subluxation and dislocation of the hip in stillborn and newborn infants. *J Bone Joint Surg* 45A:1147-1158, 1963.
91. Takahashi, H.: A histological study of bone dynamics using the secondary osteons. *Clin Orthop Surg (Japan)* 44:391-402, 1969.
92. Talmage, R. V.: A study of the effect of parathyroid hormone on bone remodeling and on calcium homeostasis. *Clin Orthop* 54:163-175, 1967.
93. Talmage, R. V.: Calcium homeostasis—calcium transport—parathyroid action, the effects of parathyroid hormone on the movement of calcium between bone and fluid. *Clin Orthop* 67:211-223, 1969.
94. Thompson, D. E., Frost, H. M., Hendrick, J. W., and Horn, R. C.: Soft tissue sarcomas involving the extremities and the limb girdles. *Southern Med J* 64:33-44, 1971.
95. Turek, S. L.: *Orthopaedics,* 2nd ed. Philadelphia, J. B. Lippincott, 1967.
96. Turner, C. D.: *General Endocrinology,* 3rd ed. Philadelphia, W. B. Saunders, 1960.
97. Urist, M. R., Silverman, B. F., Buring, K., Dubuc, F. L., and Rosenberg, J. M.: The bone induction principle. *Clin Orthop* 53:243-283, 1967.
98. Villanueva, A. R., and Frost, H. M.: Evaluation of factors determining the tissue-level haversian bone formation rate in man. *J Dent Res* 49:836-846, 1970.
99. Weinmann, J. P., and Sicher, H.: *Bone and Bones,* 2nd ed. St. Louis, C. V. Mosby, 1955.
100. Weiss, P.: Interactions between cells. *Rev Modern Physics,* 31:449-454, 1959.

101. Wiener, N.: *Cybernetics*, 2nd ed. Cambridge, Massachusetts, M. I. T. Press, 1961.
102. Wu, K., Jett, S., and Frost, H. M.: Bone resorption rates in physiological, senile and postmenopausal osteoporoses. *J Lab Clin Med* 69:810-818, 1967.
103. Yamada, H.: *Strength of Biological Materials.* Baltimore, Williams and Wilkins, 1970.
104. Young, R. W.: Specialization of bone cells. In *Bone Biodynamics.* Boston, Little, Brown, 1964, pp. 117-139.

ANSWERS TO QUESTIONS

Unambiguous answers exist to some of these questions while to others many good ones exist. In those instances of the latter case, the author will provide examples of his own choices and will identify them with an asterisk at the end of the answer.

Chapter I

1a. Any construct in which two or more parts interact.
 b. Kidney, cardiovascular system, the AMA; a village, the welfare department, the city charter; the solar system, a galaxy.*
2a. An interaction needed (directly if first order, indirectly if of higher order) for normal health and function.
 b. The organ and higher level consequences of one or more defective functions.
3. They involve direct rather than indirect interactions.
4. Bone strength matches muscle strength; pulmonary ventilation matches the state of the blood gasses; erythrocyte synthesis matches the RBC; cardiac output matches somatic need for perfusion.*
5. When diseases peculiar to one exist, it possesses functional and regulatory machinery lacking in the other.

Chapter II

1a. Skeleton: The simple tissue forms the elementary construct; adding internal structural order makes of it a complex tissue; combining either of those in any way would create other kinds of complex tissues. Various combinations of those form organs.
 b. Lung: endothelial cells, supporting tissue, alveolar epithelium; alveolus, lung.*
 c. Heart: muscle tissue, connective tissue, endothelial tissue, cardiac muscle, heart.*
2. Rickets affects growing cartilage of epiphyseal plates; adults have synostosed their plates.

236 *The Physiology of Cartilaginous, Fibrous, and Bony Tissue*

3. Chondrogenesis: creation of new skeletal tissue; special modes of response to STH and mechanical force.
   Fibrous bone: creation of new skeletal tissue; special modes of response to endocrine and mechanical factors.
   Lamellar bone: anisotropic mechanical strength and rigidity in tension, compression, and shear.
4. Two: ENOS and bone formation in membrane.
5. One can grow without modeling, but modeling cannot occur normally without growth. Both characterize the prematuration stage of life.
6. Creation must come first.
7. A very complex and subtle "musical score" derives from a very simple elementary alphabet.

Chapter III

1. Two.
2. Involved in blood-bone exchange and in the repair of mechanical microdamage.
3. Fibrous and lamellar bone; hyaline and fibrocartilage; fibrous tissue.
4a. Two: chondrogenesis, fibrous bone production.
  b. For compacta, three; for spongiosa, three; for epiphysis, one; for apophysis, one; for tendon insertion, one; for articular cartilage, one; for epiphyseal plate, one. Total: eleven.
  c. By endochondral ossification, by bone formation in membrane, and by a combination of the two. Total: three.
5. Provides anisotropic strength and rigidity in tension, compression, and shear (first-order); aligns its grain in the most effective direction (second-order); provides reservoir for blood-bone exchange.*
6. The former has derepressed the operon responsible for making chondroitin sulfate B, the second for C, and the latter for hyaluronic acid. The first two also make A, the latter does not.
7. No primary malignant neoplasm of lamellar bone osteoblasts occurs. Thus, the bony tissue in the lesion should be benign.

Answers to Questions

Request consultation with another pathologist concerning the soft tissue parts of the lesion.

8. It permitted replacement of one tissue by another kind, remodeling, and thus repair of mechanical fatigue, thus, a moderate-sized skeleton to endure with very high reliability for 100 years or so of constant use.

Chapter IV

1. The first applies to production of a simple tissue; the second to a whole bony organ such as the femur.
2. Three (the third represents the combination, as in the mandible and clavicle).
3. One each.
4. Fibrous bone, fibrous tissue. Simple elements should evolve before, not after, their complex combinations.*
5. No one knows, but it seems a particular property of the tissue.
6. *Systemic* factors include endocrine, nutritional. *Microenvironmental* ones include biomechanical and indirect effects of systemic regulation acting directly on neighboring tissues. Inherent ones represent the response characteristics determined by the genetic endowment.* Or, population dynamic; biochemical; spatial.*
7. Hyaline cartilage does not normally grow after maturity (that is why longitudinal growth ceases then). When it resumes in an adult that means the tumor tissues no longer respond to the factors normally suppressing chondral growth in adults. Suspect a low grade chondrosarcoma and obtain pathological consultation.
8. Treat her with antibiotics as though she did have it. The bone tissue needs some two to four weeks to evolve enough changes to appear detectably on an x-ray.
9. With no other evidence than that, it would be most foolish to assume that effects on the epiphyseal plate alone explained the findings; no logician worthy of the name would accept such an argument.*

238   *The Physiology of Cartilaginous, Fibrous, and Bony Tissue*

Chapter V

1. All paths and relay routes that connect anything in the diagram to ENOS could influence it.
2. Proliferative–differentiative, biochemical, and spatial polarizing factors.
3. Proliferation–differentiation; matrix synthesis–mineralization; partial replacement with fibrous bone, and then by lamellar bone.
4a. Longitudinal growth; limb and tendon insertion alignment; joint architecture.*
 b. Creation; cartilage production.*
5. Growth-related activities usually behave differently than adult-related ones under identical circumstances. Thus, no assurance or even probability exists that changes in the growth-dependent metaphyseal phenomena would help to solve diseases of adults.
6. The chondroblast division caused by STH does not form a biochemical problem in the classical and solution-chemical sense.

Chapter VI

1. The drag or shear on the capital femoral epiphyseal plate as the hip moves during weight bearing exceeds that during swing phase, and directs the epiphysis rearward; because some systemic problem has made the tissues in the region of the plate mechanically softer than normal and thus more susceptible to creep, it moves rearward.
2a. Biomechanical guidance of local articular chondral growth potential turned up by STH.
 b. Biomechanical guidance of epiphyseal plate alignment, with an assist from the articular cartilage.
3. Biphasic curve; growth faster in tension than compression; time-averages mechanical forces and resultants.
4. They lie at the complex tissue level and via the various cause-effect relays shown in Figures 5.01 and 10.02 extend all the way up and down into the system.

5. These factors somehow determine the shapes of the skeletal anlages, the spatial contributions and alignment of the musculature, and the patterns of neural integration that control them. All act as *initial conditions* and *forcing functions* which, in conjunction with the response characteristics directly granted skeletal tissues by their genetic endowment, determine how they will respond.

Perhaps in somewhat analogous fashion, the questions, What shapes the analages? Locates muscles? Determines neural integration? have analogous answers of their own in the embryological field.*

Chapter VII

1. Excessive vertical pressure on the concave sides of the curves loads the ENOS activities in the end plates into the descending limb of the growth force-response curve, retarding their vertical growth and leading to wedging.
2a. Marked muscle weakness moves the response characteristic towards the left and thus downwards.
 b. Same answer.
 c. Same answer.
 d. I do not know the answer to this one!
3. This relates to the relative chondral growth rate.
4. The greatly increased side-to-side "whip" on the knee during growth loads its condyles over into the descending limb of the response characteristic curve, retarding their vertical growth relative to the proximal and distal ends of the collateral ligaments.
5a. Probably extrinsic causes or transient intrinsic ones in the former, but permanent intrinsic ones in the latter.
 b. One must proceed more aggressively in the second group and will have to treat the child until growth ends.
 c. In the latter group you almost surely will not end up with a normal foot.

240 *The Physiology of Cartilaginous, Fibrous, and Bony Tissue*

Chapter VIII

1. The muscle's contractile force, or the "whip" on the joint.
2a. The stretching loads it carries.
 b. Look for the cause of abnormally low mechanical forces acting on it.
3a. The mechanical loads placed on it by normal function.
 b. Mechanical fatigue represents breakage or rupture under repeated loads. Muscle fatigue equates to tiring and developing progressively weaker contractions. Thus, the same word serves in two totally different contexts.
4. The tissue remodeling mechanism for both.
5. Another posterior tibial tendon lies in there somewhere and you must find it, or you have incorrectly identified it in the first place. Check the first, and if you identified it correctly look for the other one.
6. Without biomechanically competent cells in it (and no *free* graft can have such; they are infarcted), it cannot react to and correct mechanical fatigue processes.

Chapter X

1. Look at the x-rays of victims to locate the anatomical abnormalities, and biopsy those regions (which in this disease represent articular and vertebral end-plate cartilage primarily).
2. The proposal displays such ignorance of the skeletal system that the student needs a lot of help (and study) to come up with a proposal much less obviously slated to waste his time and the taxpayers' money.*
3. The possible explanations of the increased protein turnover in the intact body include far more explanations that do not require enhancement at the cellular level than those which do. In other words, without prior knowledge that the problem under study is relevant, the odds stack heavily against success. (In fact, such studies have not explained the problem, which tetracycline labeling studies in bone indicate

unambiguously arises from an increased fraction of the cells participating in protein catabolism and anabolism. The same holds true for STH and testosterone.)
4. Incredible as it may seem, several companies currently do exactly that, which *proves* the seriousness of the communication barrier in this whole field. An analogously silly procedure would constitute evaluating the bacterial effectiveness of new antibiotics by their effect on freezing points in solution.
5. Psychogenic: A metatarsal callosity proves heavy use of the foot over previous time, which becomes incompatible as an anatomical fact (in view of the order of time involved) with the marked disability manifested during the examination.*

GLOSSARY

Anisotropic: Not the same in all directions.

Bone: The word appears in many different contexts, usually unspecified. Thus various authors and disciplines may use it in a generic sense, or to signify the skeleton, or a single bony organ of pre- and/or postnatal level development, or bony tissues as a material, or to mean fibrous bone or woven bone.

BMU: Basic multicellular unit of bone modeling (which exhibits two different kinds of BMU) and bone remodeling (which has only one kind of BMU). Strong analogies exist between bone BMU, renal nephrons, lung alveoli, and glandular acini.

Chondroclast: A cell resorbing calcified cartilage.

Compliance: The readiness with which a material yields or with which a structure "gives" under the influence of an applied external force.

Compression: Pushing together or squeezing.

Control system: Any arrangement which controls the time-related behavior of any system or machine.

Creep: A very slow yielding or flowing of a structural material under an applied external load.

Cybernetics: That branch of science (and mathematics) which deals with the design and properties of control systems.

Dendritic property: That of progressively more and more numerous roots as one passes downwards through the system's vertical organizational scheme.

Differentiated: A cell which has put aside the capacity to undergo cell division and has replaced that with some particular biochemical activity which fulfills requirements of other parts of the body (examples: fibroblasts, osteoblasts, hepatic cell, muscle cell).

Disease: A malfunction which causes a significant (rather than trivial) impairment of system performance.

Fatigue: In the mechanical sense, a structural weakening arising from applied loads which nevertheless never exceed the strength of the material as determined by laboratory testing. *Fatigue failure:* A structural failure arising from fatigue-induced weakness.

Feedback: Routing information about the behavior of the system back to the facilities which control that behavior.

Formation: In this text, the manufacture of new extracellular organic matrix.

Function: Some action or property supplied by one part to another part of the system or to the intact system. The term implies purpose.

Germinal layer: A planar region in cartilage tissue within which chrondroblast division occurs and to which that division is substantially confined.

Histogenesis: The morphological processes, events, and structures involved in the creation of simple tissues, complex tissues, and organs.

Isotropic: The same in all directions.

Load: In the mechanical sense, a force applied to a material from without.

Mesenchymal cell: In this text, the progenitor, pluripotent, or stem cell which, upon receiving appropriate instructions from its microenvironment, will produce new, differentiated cells.

Modeling: In this text, the sculpting or architecturally oriented cellular activity which determines the gross architectural features of the skeleton and maintains them in a proportional sense throughout intrauterine life and postnatal growth. We distinguish chondral modeling—which relates to longitudinally acting growth processes—from bone modeling—which relates to transversely acting ones.

Negative feedback: A control system arrangement in which information about the output of the system fed back to its input acts in such a way as to correct any error in the output behavior.

Osteoblasts: A differentiated cell that makes bone, derived from mesenchymal cells. One must specify whether of the fibrous or the lamellar type.

Osteoclasts: A cell which resorbs bone of either type.

Osteocyte: A cell residing in small holes in the bone; originally an osteoblast entrapped by the organic matrix it secreted.

Relative growth rate: Growth expressed in some such terms as the period of time required to double the size of the structure at the given rate of growth.

Remodeling: Used in this text in the sense of turnover, that is, removal of older material and replacement with exactly or nearly equal amounts of newly produced material.

Resorption: The removal by osteoclasts or chondroclasts of the mineralized organic matrices of bone and cartilage.

Resultant: In the mechanical sense, that direction representing the average of all of the mechanical forces acting on the parts. The resultant may be *instantaneous,* representing the sum of all of the forces acting at a given moment, or it may be *time-averaged,* representing all of the moment to moment resultants averaged over some period of time, which one must usually specify.

Rigidity: The capacity of a material, when not subjected to excessive external loads, to maintain its own shape without taking a permanent set or deformation.

Shear: A sidewise slippage of one layer of material on another.

Strain: The physical deformation of a material under the influence of a mechanical load.

Stress: In the mechanical sense, this represents the intermolecular resistance or force that limits the deformation of a material by an externally applied load.

Subsystem: Any part of a system which possesses the same property of internal interaction.

System: Any construct in which two or more parts interact with each other.

Systems analysis: Studying a system so as to relate structure, behavior, purpose, and cause/effect in some kind of construct that has meaning from the systems control capability viewpoint.

Systems atlas: Any abstract construct, such as a diagram, map, or flow chart, which delineates those cause-effect chains in a system that determine its health, and aberrations of which determine its diseases.

Systems control capability: The ability to diagnose, prevent, and correct the malfunctions/diseases of a system.

Tension: A pulling apart.

Turnover: See remodeling.

INDEX

A

Achondroplasia, 118
Activation, 52
Adhesive, natural, 156
Adrenalcortical steroids, 41, 61
Albers-Schonberg disease, 116
Alignment, joint, 130
Alphabet, skeletal, 23-41, 44-47
Analytical inversion, 145
Androgens, 61
Ankle, 138
　ball-socket, 137
Articular cartilage, 32
Articular incongruity, 130, 136
Associative property, 193

B

Ball-socket joint, 134, 137
Biomechanics; see cartilage, bone, fibrous tissue
Biomechanical response, cartilage, 125; fibrous tissue, 168
BMU, 214
　bone: *see* fibrous bone, lamellar bone
　bone, composition of, 47
　bone drift: see drift
　bone formation rate, 222
　bone modeling: see modeling

C

Calcification front, 60
Calcified cartilage, 112
Canaliculae, 51
Cartilage: see hyaline, fibro
Cause-effect chains, 192
Cement, biological, 156
Cementing lines, 156
Chondral growth/force
　response characteric, 120-139

Chondral modeling, 120-139
Chondroblast, 64, 110
Chondrocyte, 64
Chondroitin sulfates, 49, 76
Chondromalacia, 39
Chondroosseoid, 77, 79
Chondrosarcoma, 111
Clonal level, 215
Collagen, 49
Compacta, 32, 95
Complex tissue level, 207
Complex tissues, 25, 30
Compliance, 28
Composition of a bone, 47, 76
Compression force
　on cartilage, 128, 158
Congenital hip, 140-143
Control system, 11
Coxa vara, 152
Creation
　skeletal, 35-37
Creep
　cartilage, 157
Creep compensatory
　mechanism, 175
Curvature rule, 172

D

Dendritic property, 192
Differentiation of cells, 48, 52
Disease
　definition, 6
　of resorption, 73
DNA, 74
Drift, 40
Dwarfism, 110

E

Ehrenfried's disease, 110
Electric field, 122

Embryology, 21
Enchondroma, 111
Endochondral ossification, 92, 103-119, 125
Envelopes, bone, 213
Epiphyseal cartilage, 32
Error, control system, 15, 130
Estrogens, 41, 61
Eunuchism, 118
Evolution, 21
Explosion, 13
Extrinsic causes of deformity, 151

F

Feedback, 12-17
Femoral head, 135
Fibrocartilage, 28, 68-69
Fibrogenesis imperfecta ossium, 59
Fibrosarcoma, 78
Fibrous bone, 28, 48-55
Fibrous tissue, 29, 69-70, 165-184
Flexure, 41
Fracture, 54
Functional entities, 18
Functions, 5-6, 8-10, 190

G

Genu valgum, 151
Genu varum, 151
Germinal layer, 109
Gigantism, 110, 118
Goal, research, 188
Growth, 37, 40
Growth hormone, 41, 61
Growth rate rules, 143

H

Heuter-Volkmann, 125
Hip, 135, 146
Histogenesis, 43-82
Hurler's disease, 118
Hyaline cartilage, 27, 63-67
Hyaluronic acid, 69

I

Idiopathic scoliosis, 152
Internal tibial torsion, 148
Intramembranous bone formation, 89
Intrinsic causes of deformities, 151

J

Jansen's disease, 118
Joints, 123

K

Knee, alignment, 131-133

L

Lacunae, 51
Lamellar bone, 29, 55-63
Liposarcoma, 78

M

Madelung's, 152
Maintenance, 38
Marfan's Syndrome, 110
Matrix, synthesis, 66
Maturation, 72
Mesenchymal cell, 48, 52
Mesenchymoma, 78
Metaphyseal dysostosis, 113
Metatarsus adductus, 151
Mineral salts, 51
Mineralization, 52
Minimum effective strain, 169
Modeling, 38, 40, 140, 215
Modeling laws, chondral, 140
Molecular sieve property, 57
Morquio's disease, 18
Mucopolysaccharides, 63
Muscle forces and chondral growth, 144
Mustof's disease, 182

N

Negative feedback, 15

O

Ollier's disease, 111
Ontogeny, 86
Organ, 46
Organ level, 207
Organization
    skeletal, 23-41, 190
Osteoblast, 56
Osteocyte, 51, 56
Osteoid, 50, 59
Osteoid seam, 59
Osteosarcoma, 54

P

Parathyroid hormone, 191
Parosteal osteosarcoma, 54
Pathological range, of forces, 125
Pes planus, 152
Physiologic range of forces, 125
Plumbism, 118
Population dynamics, bone cell, 224
Postmenopausal osteoporosis, 217
Posttraumatic osteodystrophy, 162
Positive feedback, 12
Primary spongiosa, 32, 114

R

Remodeling, 178, 215
Repair, 39, 176
Replacement, 37
    of fibrous by lamellar bone, 53
Research strategy, 185
Resorption, 45, 70-74
Rickets, 113

S

Scar, 177
Scurvy, 118

Secondary spongiosa, 32, 95, 115, 116
Shear, 128, 153
Sigma, 127
Simple tissues, 25, 26, 45
Spastic rocker bottom foot, 152
Spatial polarization, 80
Spongiosa, histogenesis, 115
Spontaneous fracture, 39
Strategy, research, 185
Stretch-creep rule, 173
Stretch-hypertrophy law, 168
System, definition, 5, 189
Systems analysis, 6-8
Systems atlas, 199
Systems control capability, 189

T

Talipes equinovarus, 152
Tendon callus, 177
Tendon insertion, 32
Tension force
    on cartilage, 128, 161
    on fibrous tissue, 166
Tetracycline labeling, 59
Thyroxine, 41, 61
Time averaging property, 126, 169
Time lag, 15
Tissues, 45
Trabecular bone: see primary, secondary
    spongiosa
Triple surface system, 213
Trivia, 198
Tropocollagen, 49
Turnover
    cartilage, 155

W

Woven bone: *see* fibrous bone

21⁰⁰